PROTECTING AMERICA
Exploring a New Appreciation for Our Public Health System

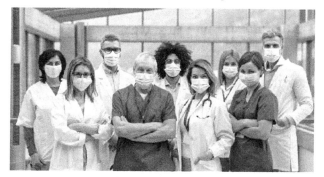

McKENNA FRIDYE, EDITOR
commentary by
Bob Kieserman and Elizabeth Linden

To request permissions, contact the publisher at powerofpatient@gmail.com

Paperback: 9798861890496

First paperback edition: October 2023

Printed by MedFocus Publications
in the United States of America

The National Library of Patient Rights and Advocacy:
The Power of the Patient Project

Cherry Hill, New Jersey 08002
www.thepowerofthepatient.org

TABLE OF CONTENTS

Foreword

The commentaries in this book are the work of a talented team of dedicated public health advocates and writers who recognize the new awareness that Americans have about our public health system. Before COVID, very few people in the country truly understood the importance and impact of the public health system. However, once the pandemic began, all of us gained a new appreciation for the many issues that our public health system addresses. We gained a new understanding of the CDC and public health warnings and protocols, and we gained a new appreciation for the important work that is done each day by our American public health system.

I have had the great privilege of editing this compilation of short essays and I have found them to be incredibly insightful. I look forward to sharing them with you, the reader.

This book provides insights on the current issues in public health. Public health is a subject that concerns every human being on earth, and is a global effort. Every country in the world has a public health initiative. Therefore, it is important for all of us to be educated about the current issues and dynamics of public health, and through this book, you will learn why. The book also offers ideas for change that we believe are very much needed. So, join us as we explore.

- McKenna Fridye, Editor
Editor

PART ONE: INTRODUCTION

Many books and many articles have been written about our public health system. Surprisingly, until very recently, very few people actually knew that much about its role and purpose. Perhaps, folks knew it existed, but did not pay too much attention to it. Actually, prior to COVID, the average American thought they had no connection to public health.

Certainly, people heard about the issues; the challenges of keeping the air quality and water quality up to standards, making sure that everyone has access to healthy food, that every American has equal access to healthcare, that homelessness is eliminated, that reproductive rights are guarded, that substance abuse is addressed, as well as other issues, but basically most folks did not equate these issues with public health, and in many cases, unless they were directly affected, most Americans paid little attention to the issues. Somewhere in Washington, D.C., these issues were being managed, and many Americans were fine with that and left it up to the government.

However, in March 2020, that all changed, and Americans as well as people throughout the world suddenly became very familiar on a daily basis with the importance and management of public health systems, as we stood by our radios to learn about the latest updates on the pandemic and learned about updated protocols sanctioned by the authorities. We became familiar with people like Dr. Anthony Fauci and CDC Director Dr., Rochelle Walensky. A new awareness arose, and most Americans became very conscious of what our public health system was all about.

We are Part of a Global System
Our public health system in the United States is part of an international network of public health systems. Almost every

country in the world has some type of public health system. In the United States, the public health policy and initiatives begin with the Department of Health and Human Services (HHS). The President appoints a Secretary of Health and Human Services to oversee this division of the federal government, and those who carry out the policies and iniatives are members of the Public Health Commission Corps, under the direction of the Surgeon General of the United States, who is always a physician. Members of the Corps are part of the uniformed services of the United States.

One of the major branches of the public health system is the Centers for Disease Control and Prevention (CDC). The purpose of our public health system according to our Centers of Disease Control and Prevention (CDC) is "protecting and improving the health of people and their communities…by promoting healthy lifestyles, researching disease and injury prevention, and detecting, preventing and responding to infectious diseases. Overall, public health is concerned with protecting the health of entire populations. These populations can be as small as a local neighborhood, or as big as an entire country or region of the world."

I think it is very important, as a preface to exploring our first section on what is public health, to also provide the reader with a statement from the website of the United Nations. The UN is indeed the leading proponent of public health endeavors in the world. This statement clearly explains the role of the UN and the World Health Organization (WHO), perhaps the most important influencers of our global public health system.

"The United Nations, since its inception, has been actively involved in promoting and protecting health worldwide. Leading that effort within the UN system is the World Health Organization (WHO), whose constitution came into force on

April 7, 1948 - a date we now celebrate every year as World Health Day.

In 1948, WHO took the responsibility for the International Classification of Diseases, which has become the international standard for defining and reporting diseases and health conditions. Since its creation WHO has contributed to many historic achievements in global public health. Some of them are:

- *Antibiotics*: (1950) The great era of discovery of present-day antibiotics begins, and WHO begins advising countries on their responsible use.

- *Polio*: (1988) The Global Polio Eradication Initiative 1988 is established at a time when polio paralyzed more than 350,000 people a year. Since then, polio cases have decreased by more than 99 per cent because of immunization against the disease worldwide.

- *Smallpox*: (1979) Following an ambitious 12-year global vaccination campaign led by WHO, smallpox is eradicated.

- *Tuberculosis*: (1995) The strategy for reducing the toll of tuberculosis (TB) is launched. At the end of 2013, more than 37 million lives had been saved through TB diagnosis and treatment under this strategy.

- *AIDS, Tuberculosis and Malaria*: (2001) The Global Fund to fight AIDS, Tuberculosis and Malaria, a new partnership and funding mechanism initially hosted by WHO, is created in collaboration with other UN agencies and major donors.

- *Children's mortality*: (2006) The number of children who die before their fifth birthday declines below 10 million for the first time in recent history.

- *Heart Disease, diabetes, cancer*: (2012) For the first time WHO Member States set global targets to prevent and control heart disease, diabetes, cancer, chronic lung disease and other noncommunicable diseases.

- *Ebola virus outbreak*: (2014) The biggest outbreak of Ebola virus disease ever experienced in the world strikes West Africa. The WHO Secretariat activates an unprecedented response to the outbreak, deploying thousands of experts and medical equipment; mobilizing foreign medical teams and coordinating creation of mobile laboratories and treatment centers. In 2016 WHO announces zero cases of Ebola in West Africa, but warns that flare-ups of the disease are likely to continue and that countries in the region need to remain vigilant and prepared.

The staff of includes medical doctors, public health specialists, scientists and epidemiologists and other experts are at work on the ground in 149 countries worldwide. They advise ministries of health on technical issues and provide assistance on prevention, treatment and care services throughout the health sector.

WHO interventions cover all areas of the global healthcare spectrum. For instance, WHO intervenes during crises and responds to humanitarian emergencies. It also works to establish International Health Regulations, which countries must follow to identify disease outbreaks and to stop them from spreading. Furthermore, WHO's work helps to prevent chronic diseases and to achieve the health-related Sustainable Development Goals."

With that introduction, we begin our book by further defining public health.

- Bob Kieserman

The Importance of Public Health

by Emily Sokol, MPH

Since 2020, public health has been in the spotlight of every news station, newspaper, and social media newsfeed. However, public health encompasses so much more than COVID-19. Public health is the science and practice of improving the health of populations, and while this includes pandemic identification and response, public health is so much more. Public health is an initiative for healthy lunches in a local school district, a state-based policy to increase the safety and accessibility of bike lanes, and a nationwide vaccine campaign to prevent the flu.

Traditionally, public health is divided into five subdivisions:
- Epidemiology
- Biostatistics
- Behavioral science
- Social and environmental determinants of health
- Health policy and advocacy

What is epidemiology?
The Centers for Disease Control and Prevention define epidemiology as "the method used to find the causes of health outcomes and diseases in populations." In other words, it is the study and investigation of how disease spreads. Examples of epidemiology in action include isolating the restaurant where a food-born disease outbreak began or investigating risk factors in cancer patients. Epidemiology aims to understand how diseases start, exacerbate, and are eradicated.

What is biostatistics?

Biostatistics and epidemiology are closely related, as biostatistics helps to inform epidemiological investigation. Statistical science can help to identify when disease levels peak beyond "normal" to let public health officials know when there is a risk for an epidemic. Biostatistics is also used to understand concrete risk factors for disease and demographic factors that put an individual at great risk for disease. Analysis from biostatisticians can also support public health planning and program evaluation.

What is behavioral science?

Behavioral science is the branch of public health that aims to understand what drives individuals to certain health behaviors and how public health problems impact an individual. Common behavioral science initiatives include smoking cessation, weight loss, and exercise programs. These programs work to improve healthy behavior in individuals and prevent unhealthy behaviors from starting or continuing.

What are the social and environmental determinants of health?

Social and environmental determinants of health are non-clinical factors that impact an individual's health. Social determinants of health can include where someone lives, their access to healthy food options, and their education. These factors may not appear to impact an individual's health, but imagine the following situation: a woman is living in a rental complex that has not been updated since lead paint regulations became law. The nearest "grocery store" is a convenience mart down the street that carries mostly non-perishable food items. In this example, the woman has greater barriers to overcome to maintain and promote positive health outcomes. She has less access to healthy food options and a housing situation that might contribute to negative health outcomes. In this woman's case, her social determinants of health may impact her health outcomes.

Environmental determinants of health are similar non-clinical factors that impact a person's health, such as the community they live in. Do they live near a freeway where they are more susceptible to breathing in toxic chemicals from cars? Does their neighborhood have sidewalks for safe walking or bike lanes? When in a clean, safe, healthy environment, there are fewer barriers to good health.

What is health policy and advocacy?
Advocacy promotes positive public health policies at the state, local, and federal levels. These policies can include traditional public health practices such as mandatory vaccination for all school-aged children and mandatory insurance coverage for preventative health screenings. However, these policies can also be more nuanced, tackling environmental, social, and political issues that impact an individual's health.

Understanding Public Health

by Maia Signore

The public health industry is responsible for providing healthcare services to individuals with different backgrounds, experiences, and medical histories. For many people, their experiences with trauma can significantly impact their overall health and well-being. Trauma-informed care is an approach that recognizes the prevalence of trauma in individuals' lives and ensures that healthcare providers are equipped to address their patients' individual needs. "Trauma-informed care shifts the focus from 'what is wrong with you' to 'what happened to you'" (Center for Healthcare Strategies).

There are 5 principles regarding this type of care: safety, choice, collaboration, trust, and empowerment. Making sure that physical and emotional safety is provided and addressed is the first step in trauma-informed care. So, let's talk about these 5 principles. Safety means ensuring physical and emotional safety, and this happens in common areas that are welcoming and in which privacy is respected. Healthcare providers should work towards creating physical spaces that feel safe and welcoming for patients. They should also prioritize communication that is sensitive and respectful toward patients. Communication styles must be patient-centered, they reflect empathy rather than sympathy towards them. It has been suggested that providers avoid asking closed-ended questions that may trigger anxiety in patients who have traumatic backgrounds but instead encourage open-ended conversations that allow patients to share at their own pace. Choice is when an individual has control, and this is where they are provided a clear and appropriate message about their rights and responsibilities. Collaboration is coming up with decisions with the individual while sharing "power," they are given a specific role in planning services for themselves. Providers should involve patients in decision-making about their own care plans and make sure they understand all aspects of their treatment options. Trust is where we would develop interpersonal boundaries with the patient and provide some sort of consistency and task clarity with them so nothing is confusing or stressful. And lastly, empowerment. This is where we would prioritize skill building and provide a setting in which individuals feel validated by everyone that is helping them. These principles are extremely important in that they make the patient feel safe and honored. This approach is used widely and has seen success because of the delicate measures taken so that the individual is cared for and helped throughout their healing process.

So why is this important? Trauma-informed care is extremely important because it acknowledges the impact of past traumas on an individual's physical, emotional, mental, and social well-being. Many individuals have experienced one or more traumatic events throughout their lives, such as physical or verbal abuse, neglect, violence, loss of a loved one, damages from natural disasters, or any type of accident. These experiences can lead to significant long-term effects on both physical and mental health outcomes. The creation and use of trauma-informed care reduces negative impacts by creating a more relaxed relationship between healthcare providers and patients.

The trauma-informed care approach started in the 1970s when the Vietnam War veterans needed it the most. "Out of the study and treatment of this population came the diagnosis of Post-Traumatic Stress Disorder (PTSD), and an awareness that trauma can affect the way in which the brain, the nervous system, and the body function or malfunction" (Ohio Leadership Council). This set the tone for this type of care and has only become more effective and efficient as time goes on.

Understanding the CDC: Its History and How It Works

by Hugo Amador

Overview of the History of the CDC

The Communicable Disease Center (CDC) was established on July 1, 1946. Having been founded on a mission to prevent the spread of malaria, the health organization has helped stand up and mitigate a variety of public health challenges around the nation since its inception. As the CDC founder made his way to the south, which at the time was the heart of the malaria outbreak, Dr. Joseph Mountain began advocating for extending the organization's outreach to other communicable diseases. Since then, the CDC has hence been called the Centers for Disease Control and Prevention.

Although epidemiologists during the 1940s were not as profound around the United States as they are today, public health became the crux of the CDC's initiatives. Many significant accomplishments such as the war against HIV, Ebola, and the eradication of smallpox, succeeded the organization's humble origins as a small organization. Especially since the start of the Covid-19 pandemic in 2020, the CDC has been in the spotlight as one of the major and best-known operating bodies within the Department of Health and Human Services. With such a prominent presence and role that the CDC plays during public health crises, it is important to know and understand how the premier public health organization works, and how its mandates influence the health of the American Public. Here is what you need to know.

How the CDC Works - An Overview of Its Structure

Considering how vast the organization has grown since its inception, with more than a dozen centers nationally, many labs, thousands of employees, and an infinite scripture of initiatives, the organization upholds the necessary structure and organization it needs to grasp public health issues. The CDC has a workforce of about 20,000 employees across at least sixty countries. These employees all follow the directorship of the organization which is typically a political appointment by the president of the United States. The director of the CDC that is appointed is always a healthcare professional— Rochelle Walensky, for example, is a medical doctor and virologist that was appointed head of the health organization through the Biden Administration transition of the presidency.

Within the last seven decades, the organization has expanded its cause in preventing and alleviating many forms of communicable and non-communicable diseases alike. Since then, the CDC has been divided into institutes, offices, and centers–there are twelve major units and more than two dozen in all–each with its focus on certain public health challenges around the nation. The Center for Injury Prevention and Control helps tackle drug overdose and suicide prevention, for example.

In times of dire public health emergencies, there is communication within the necessary centers located at the local and regional levels that respond to the federal department. Certain public-health emergencies that are pinpointed at regional levels are communicated to health departments, which are then reported to the CDC Once there, the organization can instigate specific, local guidelines in addition to federal response efforts. All these efforts depend on communication from the local regions, receptive understanding from the regions in question, and how much funding the C.D.C. has to support these responses.

How its Decisions and Mandates Positively Affect the American Public

With the rise of novel diseases, the CDC required researchers in centers that could offer relevant conclusions and applicable policies for the public based on epidemiological and public health modeling. In 1984, Congress authorized the Prevention Research Centers (PRC) within the CDC. These centers established a network of 26 research centers that identify public health emergencies and further develop, test, and evaluate public health interventions that can be applied universally–particularly in underserved communities. By documenting behavior and health outcomes in populations, the organization can manage guidance on sociologic and scientific implications.

Amid the Covid-19 pandemic, the CDC undertook testing, isolation, and vaccination initiatives, using population data collected in SARS-Cov-2 hotspots to issue guidance and mandates. Albeit not faced without skepticism, the CDC uses pertinent patient data to employ its public health policies, primarily with Covid-19. Guidelines, restrictions, and regulations that the CDC imposes from the statistics they receive matter; behind each statistic is not a number, but rather the health of a person, and the health of people around them. With trends, statistical modeling, and scientific research/data, the organization predicts the necessary restrictions needed to hinder a worsening outbreak.

For years the organization has taken the stage mainly during public health emergencies. For many health professionals, the CDC is the gold standard for national health agencies. The organization has consistently worked in tandem with the World Health Organization, in the hope of collaborating on international health emergencies. Thus, the CDC has garnered a high reputation in many parts of the world. "Quietly and effectively, the CDC projected American competence and leadership," said Sudip Parikh, chief executive officer of the American Association for the Advancement of Science.

As the Covid-19 pandemic slowly wanes in the backdrop of American life, many celebrate the freedoms that testing and vaccination efforts have revitalized–efforts invigorated through CDC support and guidance. During a global pandemic or not, the CDC consistently manages the health of the American people, in the hope of alleviating the impacts diseases impose on our well-being. Whether it be obesity, depression, diabetes, the Flu, or Covid-19, the public health organization established through the vision of Dr. Mountain is there to guide us on the relevant science and policies.

PART TWO:
PUBLIC HEALTH ADVOCACY

One of the main roles of the individuals who have made their careers public health is advocacy. These individuals are excited and determined to make others aware of how we can have a healthier lifestyle, by eating healthier food, taking better care of our elderly, promoting advancements in medicine for women, for men, for members of the LGBTQIA+ population, for children, for those who are chronically ill, and for those who are challenged by mental illness. This includes guarding the rights we have as patients and advocating on behalf of patients when the government, big business, or other entities begin to place restrictions on those rights.

These advocates are also fighting diligently on the front lines to make healthier food more available to those living in neighborhoods where healthy food is not available, while, at the same time, advocating for better and safer housing, and ending homelessness.

In this section of the book, you will also learn more about something called population health, what it is and how it affects the future of the world. We will also explore a major crisis right now – physician burnout – which has threatened the healthcare delivery system, especially in the area of maternity care.

- Bob Kieserman

Women's Health

It has only been recently that women's health has had the attention it deserves.

If you've ever sat in a doctor's office and felt like your worries or aches weren't being taken seriously—or were even dismissed—you're not alone. Women's pain and medical issues are often chalked up to normal health issues and are still often misdiagnosed as something less critical.

Whether its heart disease labeled as anxiety, an autoimmune disorder attributed to depression, or ovarian cysts chalked up to "normal period pain," the reasons for the lack of knowledge and equitable care go back literally thousands of years. Maybe longer.

Back in Ancient Greece, men believed a woman's uterus could wander through her body, causing symptoms wherever it landed. Though we now know that's far from fact, this early misdiagnosis—whether it was misogynistic or not—generated a word that has plagued women ever since. Women's mysterious ailments were diagnosed as "hysteria," derived from *hysteria*, the Greek word for uterus. Since then, many women have been called hysterical or have been otherwise gaslighted in the medical community in one way or another.
According to Elinor Cleghorn (2021) from Time magazine, while states are expected to uphold modern medicine's principle of impartiality and that women deserve fair and ethical treatment, this is not the still often not the case.

According to the National Institutes of Health (NIH), women's health in the United States has been grossly underfunded when compared to men's health. According to an article published in Northwell Health it was often the norm for male researchers to publish articles using only male subjects, whether they were animals or humans. As a result, many women went untreated or were misdiagnosed for diverse and even deadly diseases such as COPD, autoimmune diseases as these diseases present differently in women.

In response to past and current discrimination, the women's health movement focused on sexual health and abortion, and quickly progressed to other areas of concern such as doctor's dismissal of pain symptoms in women. In the 1980s and 1990s political and nonprofit organizations achieved gains for women in federal policy such as the inclusion of women in drug trials, recognition of violence against women and the development of new types of contraception. A new issue that is receiving much attention is the period desert, the inability for women in underserved populations to get access to personal products that are needed at the time of their menstrual cycle. Many communities across the country are trying to address this issue with programs focused on women's health and hygiene.

Although there have been strides to improve the issues women face, the intentional or unintentional biases women face are still prevalent.

In this section of the book, you will learn more about the current health disparities women face, the societal impact, and what women and health care providers are doing to advocate and provide equitable treatment for all.

- Elizabeth Linden

Invisible Battles: The Medical Gaslighting of Women and the Silencing of Their Pain

by Elizabeth Linden

Introduction

In Toronto, a woman named Alisa Gayle suffered from excruciating pain in her head for two years. She thought her head was going to explode and she had difficulties hearing out of her left ear. She would also run out of breath, have dizzy spells, and suffer from frequent nausea. Fatigue and exhaustion were her frequent companions. Gayle saw her family doctor in 2012. Alisa's doctor told her that her symptoms were related to excessive earwax and panic attacks. He also diagnosed her with bipolar disorder based on her previous hospitalization at the age of 16 with depression. He referred Gayle to a psychiatrist who then prescribed Seroquel which is used to treat schizophrenia, bipolar disorder, and depression. The medicine was not only ineffective, it made her sleep for days. She went back to the doctor and asked for a CT scan and other diagnostics because her pain had not subsided. Her doctor declined her requests stating she didn't need them. He was convinced all her symptoms were related to her deteriorating mental health although her complaints pertained to pain. Even though she felt fine mentally, she started to believe him. She started to believe that her mental health must be deteriorating. He was the doctor, after all. Then in 2014, she was at a baseball game and she had a seizure. When she woke up in the ER, a doctor stood over and with a puzzled look he asked, "Did you know you have a giant brain tumor?"

If Alisa's initial complaints and requests were taken seriously, she wouldn't have lost two years of her life to needless pain and worry. Maybe the tumor wouldn't have grown in her brain. She may have been saved from having to go through a 10-hour-long brain surgery. Perhaps she would have been spared from the difficult recovery that included learning to walk again and over nine years of facial paralysis that still lingers.

Like many other women, Alisa Gayle's reported symptoms were all chalked up to signs of a mental health disorder. Her requests for more diagnostics were dismissed. The source of her pain was not investigated or treated.

Dismissal of symptoms by a trusted doctor can have devastating effects both emotionally and physically. What happened to Gayle (whether done intentionally or not) is often referred to as medical gaslighting.

What is Medical Gaslighting?
Stacey E. Rosen, senior vice president for Northwell Health's Katz Institute for Women's Health, defines medical gaslighting as "when concerns about your healthcare are being dismissed, they're not heard and they are minimized."
Medical gaslighting is not a new phenomenon and it is more common to happen to women than men. The history of medical gaslighting can be seen in ancient Greece who attributed many of women's health problems stemming from problems of some sort of defect of their uterus which they believed wandered throughout the body. It's no coincidence that the word "hysteria" is derived from the ancient Greek word for "uterus." Hysteria was a common medical diagnosis for a variety of emotions or behaviors thought to be

inappropriate. The diagnosis hysteria and the notion that the uterus is the cause of many ailments are still embedded in our culture and medical community. Have you ever been angry and been told you were being 'hysterical'? Have you ever been upset or angry and asked if you were on your period?

How Often Does Medical Gaslighting Occur to Women

Pfizer and SHE Media conducted a comprehensive research study with 1,500 participants in 2022 and found that 72% of the female respondents reported that they had experienced medical gaslighting. Seventeen percent of women said that they felt they had to "prove" their symptoms to doctors or had their symptoms been dismissed. While symptoms such as pain after an injury can be inferred by a doctor, the level of pain is a personal experience. Furthermore, if the cause of the pain has not been found, the doctor relies on self-reported symptoms using a Visual Analogue Scale. When assessing symptoms, nearly 2/3 of surveyed women have been told by their doctor that their symptoms were due to stress or anxiety. Another 53% reported they were told that they needed to lose or gain weight to get better.

Can Doctors See Your Pain?

While (if allowed a CT scan as originally requested), Alisa may have received treatment before her tumor grew to the size that made recovery so difficult. The doctor would have been able to see the cause of her pain. However, it is also widely known that some pain cannot be seen through CT scans as the science is just there. Many people suffering from excruciating headache pain may show no signs of brain injury. Such is the case with Jaime Sanders. Jaime is a chronic migraine sufferer who wrote about her account of medical gaslighting in an article titled: *Finding Migraine Care: Cultural Humility and Medical Gaslighting*. The article describes her degrading experiences with a neurologist who told her she was relying too heavily on her abortive medications. Without the understanding that not all patients have the same level of pain or frequency, the neurologist implied that Jaime was lazy and unwilling to do what was necessary to get better. She goes on to explain her experiences at an urgent care facility where she would seek acute, unmanageable pain. She recalls the doctor looking visibly annoyed when she came in for the third time. The doctor asked Jaime why she would come into urgent care for a migraine. He didn't seem to comprehend that her level of pain could reach the point of what would be considered unmanageable. He dismissed her claims and appeared to have incomplete knowledge of the spectrum of migraine sufferers. In other words, he didn't believe her self-report. Given that she had been scrutinized by this same urgent care facility in the past, Jaime would come into the facility with a binder of her treatment plan in hopes of not being dismissed during future visits. This tactic backfired in a sense as the care team mocked the binder, leaving her feeling silly for having brought it. However, when the physical exam started, they would make her go through every treatment she received in the past and present before they would proceed with any treatment, regardless all while she was in excruciating pain. It was as if they expected her to remember two years of treatments that had changed over time and could articulate it while in so much pain. Furthermore, they eventually took the very binder they previously laughed at and looked at it before finally administering treatment.

Why Does Medical Gaslighting Occur?
Certainly, not every doctor would consciously ignore a patient's symptoms. The doctor or hospital can face severe consequences for dismissing a patient's symptoms if such dismissal leads to future harm. So why does medical gaslighting continue to occur in the first place?

One reason medical gaslighting occurs is that much less is known about women's bodies because they have been largely excluded from medical research until the 1990s. Men and women have biological differences and their symptoms present differently for many serious illnesses including heart disease. Assuming that men can represent the human species was a seriously flawed assumption that has hurt women.

Another reason why gaslighting continues to occur is that medical research funding continues to favor men. More money is spent researching diseases thought to be male regardless of the disease burden. For just one example of many, migraines, headaches, and anxiety disorders that disproportionately affect women attract less funding than conditions that affect primarily men. Classically considered a man's disease, coronary heart disease is now the leading cause of death of women in the United States. As women have not been equally represented in studies, the opportunity has been lost to learn how symptoms may differ. This lack of inclusion has had devastating effects such as in the case of Jenneh.

Jenneh was diagnosed with two congenital heart conditions but had been doing well for some time. Then she started to have intense chest pains that woke her in the middle of the night. She started passing out so many times that she had to use a wheelchair. When she went to a well-known cardiologist, she remembers him saying "People who have these heart conditions aren't this sick." He prescribed her two new medications but did not want to pursue the cause of the chest pains and fainting. Fortunately for Jenneh, she still felt something was off and went to another cardiologist. There she discovered that she had been having mini-heart attacks. Two months later she had open-heart surgery that probably saved her life.

There is also another form of medical gaslighting that continues which can't be wholly explained away as a result of lack of medical knowledge due to biased medical testing. Research published by the Academy of Emergency Medicine showed a disturbing pattern when it comes to emergency care for women. The data showed that women with stomach pains waited 33% longer than men who had the same symptoms. Women who had chest pains also waited longer and were also less likely to receive cardiac testing. In addition, women were less likely to receive ICU treatments for diseases regardless of the severity.

The Costs of Medical Gaslighting
Like Jaime Sanders, others have experienced emotional turmoil to the point that they find themselves in a place of distrust of the medical community. Due to the medical gaslighting similar to the experiences of the ladies mentioned above, some women are hesitant to go to the doctor at all. A survey of 12,000 European patients showed that receiving a misdiagnosis of a psychological illness can make a proper diagnosis of a rare disease take 14 times longer. Medical gaslighting that leads to delayed response time can mean more medical expenses for the individual and insurance companies. Worse yet, it can and has cost lives.

Steps You Can Take
If you feel that your doctor is downplaying your symptoms, dissuading you from researching your diagnoses, telling you that a second opinion isn't needed, or denying access to your

medical records, *Psychology Today* recommends the following steps:

- Bring a support person to appointments.
- Keep a log or diary of your symptoms and concerns.
- Get as many opinions as you need. You have the right to keep searching (albeit this is not always easy based on insurance or distance to providers).
- Know that your doctor does not have all the answers and if you feel they are not listening, they may not be the best fit.
- Ask other women what providers they would recommend.

How the Pandemic Affected Cancer Screenings in Women

a statement by The Centers of Disease Control and Prevention

Editor's Note: *This statement by the CDC was published in June 2021 in the middle of the pandemic and conveys concern for a crisis that led to many undiagnosed cases of gynecological cancer.*

The total number of cancer screening tests received by women through CDC's National Breast and Cervical Cancer Early Detection Program (Early Detection Program) declined by 87% for breast cancer and 84% for cervical cancer during April 2020 as compared with the previous 5-year averages for that month.

Prolonged delays in screening related to the COVID-19 pandemic may lead to delayed diagnoses, poor health consequences, and an increase in cancer disparities among women already experiencing health inequities.

"This study highlights a decline in cancer screening among women of racial and ethnic minority groups with low incomes when their access to medical services decreased at the beginning of the pandemic, said Amy DeGroff, PhD, MPH, CDC health scientist and lead author. "They reinforce the need to safely maintain routine health care services during the pandemic, especially when the health care environment meets COVID-19 safety guidelines."

Screening declines observed in the Early Detection Program coincided with the rapid increase of COVID-19 cases in spring 2020. Factors that might have contributed to the declines during this time include screening site closures and the temporary suspension of breast and cervical cancer screening services due to COVID-19. The requirement or recommendation to stay at home and the fear of contracting COVID-19 also likely deterred individuals from seeking health care services, including cancer screening.

Published in the medical journal *Preventive Medicine*, the **study** examined COVID-19's impact on the Early Detection Program's screening services during January-June 2020.

Health equity impact:

- Declines in breast cancer screening varied from 84% percent among Hispanic women to 98% among American Indian/Alaskan Native women.

- Declines in cervical cancer screening varied from 82% among Black women to 92% among Asian Pacific Islander women.

- In April, the number of screening tests for breast cancer declined in metro (86%), urban (88%), and rural (89%) areas compared to the respective five-year averages. The decline for cervical cancer screening tests was 85% and 82% for metro and rural areas, respectively, and 77% for urban areas.

- Screening volumes had begun to recover in all groups by June 2020, the end of the observation period.

"CDC encourages health care professionals to help minimize delays in testing by continuing routine cancer screening for women having symptoms or at high risk for breast or cervical cancer," said DeGroff. "The Early Detection Program can help women overcome barriers to health equity by educating them about the importance of routine screening, addressing their concerns about COVID-19 transmission, and helping them to safely access screening through interventions like patient navigation."

concerns about COVID-19 transmission, and helping them to safely access screening through interventions like patient navigation."

How the Overturning of Roe V. Wade Affects Women's Reproductive Healthcare

by Courtney Pokallus

The ruling of Roe v. Wade was a monumental decision made by the Supreme Court in 1973. The court ruled that the right to an abortion was backed up by the Constitution which put a stop to many anti-abortion laws both federal and state. Before this ruling, abortions were illegal in 33 states and only partially allowed due to special circumstances in 13. This led to many illegal and unsafe abortions done for women who did not have access to one. "We had almost no options. You would either put yourself at risk by self-inflicting an abortion, using knitting needles, crochet needles, anything that could stop — take big black pills. There was no other option that I knew anything about" (Byllye Avery, Health Care Activist). Many women were forced to try unsafe techniques and travel to other states and countries, but others couldn't afford to go to such lengths. Not having access to abortion put so many women in situations that they were not ready for, they only had the option of receiving an unsafe abortion or giving birth to a child that they did not have the means to take care of. Knowing how this has affected women shows how important Roe v. Wade was for women's reproductive rights then and now.

Now that the ruling of Roe v. Wade has been overturned, it is safe to say that all the rights that came with it will be taken away as well. The states that will be banning or partially banning abortions are Utah, Arizona, Texas, South Dakota, Oklahoma, Louisiana, Arkansas, Missouri, Mississippi, Alabama, Georgia, South Carolina, Tennessee, Kentucky, West Virginia, Ohio, and Wisconsin. Three states also have trigger bans which means that the ban will take place about a month after the ruling depending on the state government's decision. These states are Idaho, Wyoming, and North Dakota. Iowa and Indiana are also likely to ban abortion, but the decision has not been set as of now. Although there are only 22 states banning abortion or likely to ban abortion compared to the 33 pre-Roe, this still leaves millions of women without the reproductive rights they had before the overturning.

Although abortion can be used to terminate an unwanted pregnancy, there are also other reasons for getting an abortion like treating miscarriages and ectopic pregnancies. Many know that a miscarriage is the loss of a pregnancy before the fetus is able to survive independently, but do not know what exactly an ectopic pregnancy is and how it differs. An ectopic pregnancy is when the egg is fertilized outside of the uterus, mostly in the fallopian tubes. This can cause the tube to rupture and result in internal bleeding. Ectopic pregnancies can become life-threatening to the woman and are treated with abortion. This is in the form of surgery to remove the egg or by taking medication that stops the cells from growing which terminates the pregnancy. In many of the states where abortion has been banned, it is illegal for a doctor to perform this procedure under any circumstance. This means in cases of ectopic pregnancy where it is a risk to the women's health, physicians will have to choose between being persecuted or letting their patient die.

Another issue when looking into post-Roe America is privacy. HIPAA, the Health Insurance Portability and Accountability Act, provides patient confidentiality and privacy. It protects patients by not allowing the sharing of medical documents and information but could not provide much protection in lieu of Roe v. Wade being overturned. This is because HIPAA does allow the sharing of medical information with the authorities. This could allow physicians to report a patient looking to get an abortion and ultimately end in jail time for the woman. This also does not protect against the sharing of information from period tracking apps. This means that if it looks like a woman could have had an abortion from her period tracker data, she could be persecuted as well.

The overturning of Roe v. Wade has brought a scary and unprecedented time for women living in America but knowing what could happen and other resources to help in these situations is very important. One of these resources is prochoice.org which has assets for women looking to get an abortion such as hotlines, what to expect from an abortion and where to find them, as well as resources for pregnancy. They also provide resources for physicians and providers like information on how to continue medical education on abortion. There are sites that offer abortion pills to be shipped anywhere in the United States. The FDA allows these medications to be mailed to any state by specific licensed physicians. This is crucial information for every woman to know as even though abortion is illegal in specific states, there is still a way. The Biden Administration also is looking into declaring a public health emergency to expand access to abortion in all states. They are looking at the legal authority they have to be able to declare this emergency, but there may be a way for abortion to be protected federally without Roe v. Wade.

Looking at the Current Discussion on Reproductive Rights from the Historical Perspective

by Hugo Amador

In May 2022, a Supreme Court justice clerk leaked an opinion draft that declared the Supreme Court voted to overturn one of the most talked about cases since its inception: Roe v. Wade.

In this 1973 decision, the Supreme Court deemed that individuals had a constitutional right to abortion. Roe v. Wade was grounded on the Fourteenth Amendment, which declared that individuals have a "right to privacy." However, with time, this legal argument was faced with critique against the ambiguity of the Fourteenth Amendment.

For decades after its inception, Roe v. Wade's support was padded by a historical narrative; state laws prohibiting abortion at all stages of pregnancy were not imbedded in the jurisprudence of ancient law. Rather, the restrictions were seeded in the latter half of the 19th century. Before this, abortion early in pregnancy was allowed in most states.

States like Illinois and New York were some of the first to criminalize abortion in the late 19th century. The restrictive laws were initially enacted in response to alarming claims of failed abortion attempts which, at times, would lead to death. In 1857, the newly founded American Medical Association began the wave against allowing abortion at any period of gestation. It appeared as if the organization was motivated by concern about fetal life, but also by concern that middle-class

"Anglo-Saxon" birth rates were not up to par compared to those of immigrants and individuals of color.

The new draft opinion written by Supreme Justice Alito is a complete repudiation of the 1973 decision, and likewise of the 1992 decision Planned Parenthood v. Casey which confirmed and maintained the rights enacted in Roe v. Wade.

"Roe was egregiously wrong from the start," Alito writes. "We hold that Roe and Casey must be overruled."

The draft relies heavily on originalism; it appears as if Alito's draft focuses and relies on provisions regarding federal protections for trial by jury and against self-incrimination and how it does not parallel an individual's right to abortion. This suggests that the roots of the "deep rootedness" runs in conjunction with a deeply anglophile national fantasy. The Fourteenth Amendment, in which Roe and Casey were justified, surfaced quandaries regarding the rights of individuals against the states. However, it may appear – through a peruse of Alito's precedents – that the judges did not have a bedrock for determining, objectively, which rights are not federally protected against the states.

So perhaps a history-based approach, or rather a conclusion on stare decisis, cannot be the means of defining the rights of a patient, an individual. In appealing to the national spirit of a people, more so those past rather than present, the question still depends on which people exactly? Perhaps their motivations were to rule out – in the contexts of tradition, history, and liberty – the years since Roe's rectification. And likely, perhaps, to rule out those who aren't with them on the issue as well. Many may come from the perspective that laws inhibiting individuals who become pregnant from exercising a choice of abortion, or, generally, on mitigating their own reproduction are clear violations of elements "implicit in the concept of ordered liberty," Alito and the remaining four judges do not seem to think so. There may be a difference of opinion, but theirs appear to be contoured by a deeply rooted tradition of calling the individual, the patient, the physician, not just incorrect, but completely shy of the discussion.

The fight to overturn these two cases is not a novel one. Growth in conservative perspective around the country, bolstered by a conservative administration in the last 5 years, sought many means to repeal, or hinder, women's rights to abortions in America.

In 2017, two undocumented individuals in custody sued the Trump administration for a policy against allowing abortions in detention agencies. Tens of thousands of unaccompanied, undocumented migrants are apprehended at the border each year. With many of them having suffered sexual abuse and rape in their home country or during their journey to the U.S., numerous come from countries in Central and South America that wholly outlawed abortions.

Countless undocumented women seek refuge in the U.S. partly for oppression against their rights in their home countries. Many claim that overruling Roe and Casey is entirely an attempt to return the decision on abortion to the states, though allowing women who want an abortion to travel across state lines, should they want one. However, this is not an equitable approach toward immigrant women and women in poverty who do not have equal feasibility of seeking health services in different states.

The current dilemma, therefore, can be approached from an equity point of view, rather than a historical and/or moral standpoint. As Ruth Bader Ginsburg exclaimed, regardless of whether Roe and Casey are overturned, "If you have the sophistication and the money, you're going to have someplace in the United States where your choice can be exercised in a safe manner." Thus, this would mean that poor and immigrant women would not have a choice like wealthier Americans.

Men's Health

As men and women live longer, the issue of men's health has received much more attention than ever before from the public health world. One of the great challenges that the advocates face is that men tend to be less proactive about their health than women, and many medical issues that could be addressed early and reversed are not because men tend to procrastinate in seeing a doctor. This is especially true with prostate health. Many men do not heed the warnings of the public health advocates to be tested for prostate cancer using a PSA blood test, and too often, prostate cancer is found too late. Likewise, many men walk around with elevated blood pressure as well as heart issues, and since they are not being seen by their physicians, these very manageable medical issues are not diagnosed, and many men die prematurely because of not being properly care for. The goal of the public advocates in the area of men's health is to educate and to encourage men to pay attention to their health, have annual visits to their primary physician and any specialists they need to see, and to become proactive and serious about taking care of themselves. This next section features commentaries about some of these issues.

- Bob Kieserman

Understanding the Male Life Expectancy

by Ruby Laine

The Centers for Disease Control and Prevention reports that the life expectancy for males is around 73.5 years on average. Yet, their female counterparts have a life expectancy of 79.3 years. For the first time ever, the US is experiencing drops in life expectancy. It is estimated that once Generation Z has kids, the next generation will be the first to not have higher life expectancies than their parents.

Why are life expectancies overall decreasing?

The pandemic was a significant shift for everyone, and years after the first outbreak, we still feel its impact. Covid-19 became one of the top 3 killers of Americans, only behind heart disease and cancer. Recently another public health concern has risen with overdoses and drug-related deaths. Lastly, suicide and poor mental health are among the increasing concerns for public health and life expectancies.

Why are men experiencing lower life expectancies?

Some scientists concur that many factors are contributors, such as risky behaviors, poor lifestyle habits, and even less estrogen. Men are more likely to partake in smoking and excessive drinking, they are more likely to take risks that increase their risk of life-threatening injuries, and they are less likely to visit a doctor. Men are more likely to avoid doctors in fear of receiving bad news, being seen as less masculine, or simply because it is not ingrained in them to make regular visits, unlike women and suggested OB/GYN appointments. In a study titled *The Darwin Awards: sex differences in idiotic behavior*, men are likelier to play risky sports, have dangerous occupations, and even make "stupid" decisions. Some biological reasons are also being explored, such as increased estrogen can assist in reducing harmful cholesterol related to heart disease. Women are also thought to have more robust innate immune systems and, therefore, can fight off viral infections with better protective antibodies. Men are also at the heart of the increase in suicides. On average, women are much more likely to report and seek help when struggling, but due to stigma and cultural norms, men don't receive the support they should. Another critical factor is that as you age, social connections become incredibly important for mental health and overall well-being, which tends to be a struggle for older men.

What can be done?
Doctor's appointments for check-ups or taking that initiative when something is off can save your life. Screening and prevention are necessary to stay healthy as we age. Prioritizing your mental health and asking for help if needed is crucial. Interventions working to change the stigma and current mindsets in men around care must be prioritized to see a change in life expectancy. On a more personal level, our bodies deteriorate with age; it's natural. Still, how you take care of it makes the difference. This means having a healthy and balanced diet, being physically active, drinking water, getting good sleep, having close friends, and talking about your feelings. Health is holistic, and it should be treated as such. Additionally, expanding access and treatment availability, as well as education in prevention, could all benefit and work to increase male life expectancy.

Six Important Routine Screenings Men Need to Know About

by Liya Moges

Maintaining good health is a crucial aspect of leading a fulfilling and productive life, and it is equally important for men to be proactive about their well-being. It is important to understand how receiving regular checkups can play a pivotal role in preventive healthcare. These checkups allow for the early detection and management of potential health concerns in the future and can help many men be more proactive with their health. In this article, we will explore the essential checkups that men should undergo at different stages of life to ensure their overall health and well-being.

1. Routine Physical Examinations:
Regular physical examinations provide a holistic assessment of an individual's health status. These examinations usually involve measuring vital signs, such as blood pressure, heart rate, and body mass index (BMI). A healthcare provider will also conduct a thorough physical examination, including a check of the heart, lungs, abdomen, and other vital organs. Routine checkups are important to have at least once a year for men of all ages to ensure that you (or your male family member) are growing and developing in a healthy manner, all while taking note of any health concerns one may have during the course of their lifespan. Having a consistent routine checkup can allow your providers to keep track of your health and be able to notice any changes to your health in a smooth manner.

2. Blood Pressure Screening:

Hypertension, or high blood pressure, is a common condition that can lead to serious cardiovascular complications if left untreated. Men should have their blood pressure checked at least once every two years, starting from the age of 18. If blood pressure is consistently elevated, more frequent monitoring and lifestyle modifications may be recommended. Frequent monitoring of blood pressure may be necessary if you are a male individual who participates in risk factors such as smoking, living a sedentary lifestyle, excessive alcohol consumption, high sodium intake, or if an individual has certain medical conditions such as diabetes or kidney disease. If blood pressure readings show consistently elevated levels, it is important that you take the initiative to modify your lifestyle as advised by your healthcare provider in order to prevent any future concerns or illnesses.

3. Cholesterol and Lipid Profile Testing:

Elevated cholesterol levels contribute to the development of cardiovascular diseases. Men should undergo a fasting lipid profile test starting from the age of 20, and every four to six years thereafter. Elevated levels may necessitate lifestyle changes or medication to manage cholesterol levels effectively. While these sorts of testing may not be as discussed as often, it's an important test for male individuals who have high cholesterol levels or have any additional risk factors such as a family history of heart disease, obesity, smoking, diabetes, or high blood pressure. If the lipid profile test reveals elevated levels, lifestyle modifications as advised by your healthcare provider are made to ensure your health in the future.

4. Prostate Health Evaluation:

Prostate cancer is a significant concern for men, especially as they age. The American Cancer Society suggests that men should discuss prostate cancer screening with their healthcare provider starting from the age of 50, or earlier for those at higher risk. Screening tests may include a prostate-specific antigen (PSA) blood test and a digital rectal examination (DRE). Both exams may be uncomfortable however the decision to undergo prostate cancer screening should be made based on an informed discussion between the individual and their healthcare provider, considering the individual's risk factors, preferences, and potential benefits of the screening. Regular discussions of any concerns or questions with a healthcare provider are crucial and can provide guidance on the appropriate timing and frequency of these screenings based on an individual's health history.

5. Colorectal Cancer Screening:

Colorectal cancer is the third most common cancer in men. Screening for colorectal cancer typically begins at the age of 50. Options for screening include colonoscopy, which is recommended every 10 years, or alternative tests such as fecal occult blood tests (FOBT) and sigmoidoscopy, which may be performed more frequently. These screenings aim to detect precancerous or early-stage cancerous growths in the colon or rectum and allow for timely intervention and treatment. Early detection through regular colorectal cancer screening plays a vital role in reducing mortality rates and improving overall treatment outcomes. Male individuals with a family history of colorectal cancer or other risk factors are recommended to receive more frequent monitoring.

6. Testicular Exam:

Testicular cancer is relatively rare but can affect men of all ages. Self-examination is recommended monthly to check for any lumps, swelling, or other abnormalities in the testicles. Men should consult a healthcare professional if they notice any concerning changes. It is also recommended that men perform self-exams, which can be discussed with your healthcare provider so that individuals may be able to perform and observe for themselves for any signs of concern in a successful manner. By performing regular self-exams and seeking medical attention for any concerning findings, men can increase the chances of early detection and successful treatment of testicular cancer or other test

Prioritizing regular checkups and preventive care is fundamental to maintaining optimal health as men grow older. By being proactive and vigilant about their well-being, men can identify and address potential health concerns early on, leading to improved outcomes and a higher quality of life. Note that while all screenings and exams mentioned above are important to have, many individuals differ in their situation, risk factors, and family history, so while taking all of these tests are beneficial, it's important to know which exam or screening benefit you the most based on your background. Remember, consulting with healthcare professionals and following their recommendations is vital in ensuring comprehensive care and overall well-being.

The Elderly

Aging and the caring for the elderly are two of the most important issues on which public health advocates are focused. With many people living into their nineties, many in good health, there is a new need for public health advocates to guarantee the best quality of life possible for the elderly through proactive programming. At the same time, sadly, because of aging, many of our elderly live their final years in sickness, and other public health initiatives are necessary to educate caregivers about taking care of their family members, making sure that the elderly have proper housing, regulating nursing homes and assisted living communities to make sure they are providing optimum care, and working with medical researchers to encourage medical advancements that will make the senior years good years and serene years.

This next section addresses some of the major issues in public health as they relate to aging and the elderly.

- Bob Kieserman

Healthy Aging

by Maia Signore

The World Health Organization defines healthy aging as "the process of developing and maintaining the functional ability that enables well-being in older age." Healthy aging is important because it contributes to life expectancy, and it directs whether a person has a healthy or not-too-healthy life. Ways to promote healthy aging include exercising regularly, eating a healthy diet, not smoking or ingesting other substances, managing your stress, and many more that aren't talked about as much. These main ideas guide individuals through a healthy, less stressful, and non-toxic life.

Some may ask if you get out of an unhealthy lifestyle, are you able to age healthily? That is very possible if you don't start too late. One would like to think that it is never too late, which in most cases is true, however, in order to reach the full potential of aging and living a healthy lifestyle, there does have to be some sort of timeline. For example, if you are smoking and drinking daily or don't exercise ever and you are in your twenties, thirties, or even forties, maybe even a little bit older, if you stop that daily occurrence and start watching what you eat and going to the gym regularly, you are then able to turn yourself around and reach your healthy aging potential. However, if you are in your seventies or eighties, and you realize you would like to lose weight and live healthier, it is not that it is too late, but it's late to reach your full potential. This is because that point of your life has unfortunately already passed and certain medical conditions and issues arise when you are older; that is just a general statement and fact that changing your lifestyle won't result in any difference. That is not to say they cannot reach their original goal of losing weight and living a healthier lifestyle. They can go on walks; daily physical exercise is extremely important for older individuals to do because it gets them up and moving around instead of just sitting in one place not doing any good for their bodies. Physical activity like exercise gets the blood moving and prevents or delays any future medical issues that come with age or would result from their current lifestyle. Not to mention, it develops and/or enhances muscles in their bodies that can help them not require assistance or become dependent on others to help them move or get around. Additionally, it results in weight loss from all parts of the body.

Finally, there are six components everyone should know about healthy aging. These include physiological and metabolic health, geriatric syndromes, risk factors, physical capacity, cognitive capacity, and psychological well-being. Some of these are obviously out of our control, but those in our control give a chance for individuals to live healthy and have a successful life. Aging healthy is not a privilege, it is something you either work for to gain back or you work to prevent an unhealthy lifestyle.

The Burden of Caregiving in an Aging Society

by Kylie Tangonan

Our society is aging at a pace that we have never experienced before in human history. The number of people in each age cohort who are reaching their eighties, nineties, and even hundreds is growing and will drastically change age demographics in every single country. The question at hand is: How will the world adjust to this shift in age demographics? One crucial aspect of this phenomenon that we must consider is the realm of care. Aging brings on many changes in one's functioning. Slowing, stiffness, memory challenges, and frailty are a few amongst a myriad of other diseases and disabilities that may require older people to have access to more intensive and involved care.

The Cost of Care

For older people who need care in their day-to-day lives but cannot rely solely on their family, facility-based long-term care services are an option that can provide older adults with the care and services they need to maintain their quality of life. These facilities offer a variety of services ranging from housing and housekeeping to personal care and medical services. Odds are you know someone who utilizes or lives in a care facility. Today, someone turning 65 has a 70% chance of needing long-term care, but for many families, the cost of facility-based care is out of reach. According to the 2020 Cost of Care Survey by Genworth Financial, the annual median cost of care is $106,000 or $19,240 for adult daycare services.

The Burden of Care

The cost of facility-based care leaves many families to resort to partners, relatives, friends, and neighbors to provide care for their loved ones. The caregiver can fulfill many different roles and their care can range from assisting their loved one with making doctor's appointments to transportation, monitoring their symptoms and medications, taking on household chores, providing emotional support, or other self-care tasks such as dressing or bathing. The role of caregiving is heterogeneous, and the needs of the older person can range depending on their health status, age, and overall mobility and independence. This work is often unpaid, and although family involvement in a loved one's care is not a new phenomenon, in recent years, it has become more common and much more complex. Many family members provide care for older adults while juggling their own job, families, and other responsibilities. Acting as a caregiver can be a fulfilling role, and it is often carried out from a place of love and concern for a family member. The caregiver may find that providing care instills confidence in their caregiving abilities and helps them build a relationship with the care recipient. However, the caregiving role can also be a major physical and emotional stressor for the caregiver. Negative effects include psychological distress, strained social relationships, and a decrease in overall physical health.

How do we address the burdens that come with care?

Given the range of needs and varying responsibilities of caregivers, there are many interventions that can help families provide the best care possible while also maintaining a healthy caregiving relationship. A public health approach to address family caregivers reveals a range of actions that can promote a healthier and more balanced care landscape such as:

- Educating healthcare providers on the health risks for caregivers
- Encouraging caregivers to make use of care resources, tools, and supportive programs and services to help them provide care
- Encouraging caregivers to get regular checkups and engage in self-care to maintain health and ensure access to self-management programs
- Expanding paid leave policies to provide caregivers with financial support if they need to leave work to provide essential care to a family member
- Shifting the perspective of caregiving from family members as legitimate and taxing work that should be compensated
- Expanding Medicare, Medicaid, and other insurance programs, to assist families in getting their loved ones into appropriate and high-quality long-term care facilities

Our society will continue aging into the 21st century, and care is only one aspect that we must consider amongst other major societal shifts due to demographic changes. As we prepare for our aging society, we must reconsider society's infrastructure and resources that will allow us to increase health, productivity, and access to support for both older and younger generations.

Talking about Death

by Teri Halliwell

Spoiler alert!

We don't live forever.

And people don't like to talk about death. That may be because they're young and have a sense of immortality, scared of the unknown, fear of experiencing their consciousness descending into a black abyss of nothingness, leaving their loved ones behind, or having regrets.

Society is structured around removing the dead as quickly as possible from the living. It is a topic often highlighted as macabre with a negative connotation, even though death is as natural as birth and is one thing – probably the only thing – we know it's going to happen for sure to all of us.

Even morticians make the dead look like elegant wax model replicas of their erstwhile living selves. Attendance of children at funerals and cemeteries is generally not encouraged, adding to the sense of dreaded unfamiliarity with death.

So why do we choose to distance ourselves from the inevitable? Why do we choose to close our eyes in front of a perfectly natural event and learn how to fear death and not embrace it?

For the person who is dying, Ralph Lewis, a psychiatrist at Sunnybrook Health Sciences Centre in Toronto, Canada, says our fear of dying has been generated and cultivated throughout the years of human history based on how we imagine death to be; thus, from the view of unrealistic, unfounded fears.

Let's deal first with our fear of a painful death.

We are all afraid of pain.
Physical pain arises from damage to our living tissue. Since death is the ultimate destruction of our living tissues, we naturally assume that death must be the ultimate painful experience. Since nobody who has actually died can tell us what it felt like physically, we naturally have a terror of dying.

But from a medical point of view, there is no particular reason to suppose that the intensity of pain from various causes of death is greater than the intensity of pain from various illnesses and injuries, or the pain that others have experienced and survived to tell the tale.

The process of our existence ending and our consciousness being aware of it is also part of these unfounded fears.

Medically, we are ceased, extinguished, kaput. Being dead will not feel like anything—no more so than we felt, say, a year before we were born. There simply will be no Us to do the feeling. Dr. Lewis says here that it can be hard for us egotistical creatures to imagine that the world exists independently and continue to do so after we die, and we won't be there to continue experiencing it.

And for a good reason. We have a memory of being alive, of experiencing life, and our whole lives are shaped around this concept. We cannot perceive that death will end all of this because our consciousness is programmed to live and not to die. So, our consciousness is scared that death will take this control away.

But wait. We have actually felt how it is to drift away and lose control. When we fall asleep or when we go under anesthesia. Unless we have partial awareness, like dreaming, dying is no different than falling asleep, only this time you never wake up.

For the person who watches someone else dying emotionally and physically, it can take a toll, especially if you are watching your loved one wither away.

Depending on the cause of death, the age of the person, and the fatality of the situation, acceptance is challenging. Don't be afraid to reach out for help in order to cope with your emotions.

We are emotional beings, and it is only normal for these emotions to overtake us, as normal as it is to die. If we take a look around us, we know that life is not fair. It's not perfect and not only happy – but also not only sad.

No matter what our religious beliefs are, we strive to find the meaning of what is the purpose of life. What is the meaning of being here on Earth, still, while others have departed early, abruptly, or even just on time, and we are left grieving with so many questions.

While in philosophy and religion, we may find some of these answers to our questions, medicine says having a clearer understanding of what dying looks like can help us face our own death or the death of a loved one when the time comes. And having an idea of what's to come can make us more capable caregivers as we comfort a loved one who's dying.

The LGBTQIA+ Population

The year 2022 marked the 40th anniversary since the AIDS epidemic. Patients, like Dab Garner, who was interviewed by CBS News that year, still reflects upon the horror as his life was turned upside down within days after his diagnosis in 1989. He recounts the stigma of what was called the "gay disease" and how it changed his life. While he lived after his diagnosis, his partner and child were not so lucky. Garner recollects how the lack of government protection for those afflicted with the deadly disease left people extremely vulnerable to even more misfortune. It was not uncommon for people to lose jobs and homes within 24 hours of being diagnosed with the potentially deadly disease. Almost 20 years, when Ladeia Joyce, a black woman diagnosed in 2016 was diagnosed as HIV positive, she was confused with her diagnosis as her partner was male and black. She thought, wasn't this supposed to be a gay disease? Although she dealt with shame at first, Ladeia (like many others) turned the discrimination she felt into advocacy. There is little doubt that the shame, stigma and misinformation about the disease not only led to its proliferation but also its death toll. In fact, AIDS has been more deadly than all other pandemics combined since H1N1 hit the US in 1918. Even though there are lifesaving treatments available for the disease, another 1.3million people acquired the disease in 2022.

AIDS is not the only health concern facing Ina part of the LGBTQIA+ population, nor is it confined to that population. It is just an example of how discrimination, fear and lack of medical knowledge can have not only devastating impact on the community, but for all of society.

In this chapter we will examine the current challenges facing the LGBTQIA+ population in accessing healthcare as well as how lingering discrimination and victimization continues to lead to increased physical and mental health challenges. In addition, we will examine the positive impact of non-profit groups such as NAMI and the Trevor Project that have championed for the fair and equitable healthcare treatment of LGBQTIA+ community.

- Elizabeth Linden

LGBTQ+ Patients Face Challenges in Having Equal Access to Healthcare

by Hugo Amador

Every October, the country celebrates the annual month-long commemoration of Lesbian, Gay, Bisexual, Transgender, and Queer individuals around the country. This celebration honors the 1969 Stonewall uprising in Manhattan, from which the decades succeeding it has been spent memorializing members of the community who have been lost to suicide, hate crimes, or HIV/AIDS.

The overall purpose of the recognition has been to highlight the impact the LGBTQ+ individuals have had on history locally, nationally, and internationally as well as emphasize the human rights that each individual in the community is entitled to. However, this year's pride month was met with backlash from state legislators and officials attempting to rescind certain accessibility to healthcare treatments within the LGBTQ+ community. Overall, more than 300 bills targeting LGBTQ+ rights in state legislatures, many of which aim to limit access to healthcare or promote the use of conversion therapy. These bills have been introduced even after major medical organizations such as the American Medical Association and the American Academy of Child and Adolescent Psychiatry have condemned their practice. The bills targeting LGBTQ+ patients were introduced as a comeback to the Biden Administration, which conjunctively with the Department of Health and Human Services, announced it will enforce Section 1557 of the Affordable Care Act and Title IX to prevent discrimination based on sexual orientation and gender identity.

Additionally, the Biden Administration's American Rescue Plan aims to make investments in equitable recovery, which hopes to help LGBTQ+ families across the country recover from COVID-19. These policies come after the previous administration had finalized and regulated policies that had eased protections for transgender patients against discrimination by doctors, hospitals, and health insurance companies. However, the Biden Administration is putting emphasis on the Affordable Care Act, the 2010 law that established broad civil rights protections in healthcare, banning discrimination based on race, color, national origin, sex, age, or disability.

Even with the law, transgender patients continue to face obstacles that bar them from equitable access to healthcare treatments and services. Insurance, for example, proved to be a common issue; families struggled to get puberty blockers covered, while others found it difficult to find trans-friendly providers in-network. Now with the proposed bills introduced in state legislatures, LGBTQ+ individuals fear a harder time getting proper treatment.

Let's Stop the Stigmas and Discrimination Against HIV and AIDS

by Bri Allison

HIV and AIDS carry a lot of stigmas. Since the 1980s when the HIV and AIDS epidemic started, HIV-positive people have faced immense discrimination and prejudice because of their disease. Even today, many Americans lack a basic understanding of the infections because their knowledge of HIV and AIDS is limited to misconceptions that have been around since the beginning of the epidemic. It's time we do our part to educate ourselves on HIV and AIDS so that we can raise awareness and stop the stigma.

What is HIV?

HIV stands for human immunodeficiency virus. The virus causes damage to the immune system by attacking cells that help the body fight infection, which in turn makes the person more exposed to other diseases and infections. HIV is unfortunately a lifelong disease. There is no cure for HIV, nor can the body get rid of the virus.

Is there treatment?

However, there is treatment available. There is an HIV medication called antiretroviral therapy, also known as ART, that can be prescribed to reduce the amount of HIV in the blood to a low level. When the HIV in the blood is so low that a lab can't detect the virus, the person has achieved an undetectable viral load.

So, if someone with HIV reaches an undetectable viral load, takes the medicine as prescribed, and can maintain an undetectable viral load, then they can live a long and happy life. They also will not have to worry about transmitting HIV to their HIV-negative partners through sex.

How is it transmitted?
HIV is transmitted through contact with certain bodily fluids of someone who is HIV-positive, such as blood, semen, vaginal fluids, breast milk, amniotic fluid, pre-ejaculate, and rectal fluids. The most common transmissions are during unprotected sex (sex without a condom or medicine to prevent or treat HIV) or through sharing injection drug instruments like needles or syringes.

However, there are now ways to help prevent getting HIV through sex or drug use, such as the medicine PrEP which is pre-exposure prophylaxis, or PEP which is post-exposure prophylaxis. PrEP is a medicine used as a preventative measure for people at risk of getting HIV from sex or drug use and PEP is a medicine that can be taken within 72 hours after possibly being exposed to the virus.

What is AIDS?
AIDS is acquired immunodeficiency syndrome and is the third and final stage of HIV. When a person is diagnosed with AIDS their immune system is severely damaged and at this point of the infection, they can have a very high viral load which means they can easily transmit HIV to others.

Without proper HIV medication, a person diagnosed with AIDS will typically only have 3 years left to live. Most people in the United States that have HIV don't develop AIDS because they take the HIV medication as prescribed which stops the progression of the infection.

What are the stigmas surrounding HIV and AIDS?
HIV only affects certain groups of people.
Although some people are at a higher chance of contracting HIV, the virus can be transmitted to anyone. It does not matter your gender, sexuality, or ethnicity. According to WebMD, about 1 in 6 men and 3 in 4 women who have heterosexual contact with an infected person have contracted HIV.

Misconceptions:
HIV can be transmitted through touch, or you can get it from being around someone who is HIV-positive.
No, you can't contract HIV through touch like hugging, shaking hands, or using the same equipment that an HIV-positive person has used. You can't contract it from saliva by kissing, using the same water fountain, or sharing utensils. You can't contract HIV by breathing the same air or touching their tears, urine, or sweat. The CDC has confirmed that HIV is only spread through blood, semen, vaginal fluids, breast milk, amniotic fluid, pre-ejaculate, and rectal fluids.

I could tell if my partner is HIV positive.
Someone could have HIV for years without ever knowing because they might not present any symptoms. The only way to truly know is to get tested. The CDC recommends that everyone between the ages of 18 and 64 should be tested.

HIV can only result in death.
At the beginning of the HIV and AIDS epidemic, the death rate was very high because they didn't have the necessary medicine or treatment options that we have today. Thankfully, we have the resources, such as ART, PrEP, and PEP that have drastically increased the life expectancy of those who are diagnosed with HIV. If you're HIV-positive, you can still live a long and happy life.

HIV isn't as big of a concern as it used to be.
Although HIV diagnosis and treatment have come a long way since the 1980s, it still is a global public health concern. As of August of this year, about 38 million people worldwide were diagnosed with HIV and AIDS.

The discrimination against those with HIV and AIDS
People who are diagnosed with HIV or AIDS often face discrimination and are ashamed of their diagnosis because of the prevailing stigma. Those who are living with HIV may be refused housing and healthcare services, and/or be fired from their job.

Their job could be terminated because of the increased healthcare needs that they need such as time off for doctor appointments or testing. They also might be discriminated against by their superiors or coworkers for being diagnosed with HIV. Because of their lack of employment, they may have trouble finding adequate housing. Those who are HIV-positive may also be discriminated against by their landlord or their neighbors. Lastly, they could be denied services by a healthcare provider who is not fully educated on HIV.

Their relationships can also suffer from stigma and discrimination. Someone who is HIV-positive may be subjected to bullying, rejection, and gossip, and can even experience violence from others. The misconceptions can also impact their sexual relationships.

And all these challenges, discrimination, and stigma that those with HIV have to endure impact their mental health negatively. They can even have internalized stigma about HIV. They then can struggle with their self-worth, depression, anxiety, addiction, and more.

It is important to educate ourselves on HIV and AIDS to help fight against the stigma and end the discrimination that those who have been diagnosed face. December is HIV and AIDS awareness month so there's no better time to educate, speak up, and be a part of the movement to erase the HIV and AIDS stigma.

Mental Health

Perhaps of all of the issues facing public health advocates today, one of the major goals is improving mental healthcare in the United States. Considered by many to be available only to those who can pay expensive fees to private therapists, the challenge is that millions of Americans need help and cannot afford to pay privately. The public health system is focused on finding ways to deliver quality free care to everyone who needs it through government supported and nonprofit supported mental health centers. At the same time, the public health system has the goal of reaching out to as many people as possible to screen for mental health issues. There is a great incidence of depression and suicide in the United States, and the public health system is committed to making it easier for every American to find and get quality mental healthcare at the lowest cost possible.

In the first three essays in this section, Courtney Pokallus and Alix Greenblatt explain some of the major issues America's public health advocates are facing as they try to bring about greater access to mental health care, and greater awareness of the options available to anyone who needs help.

- Bob Kieserman

The Stigma Behind Mental Health

by Courtney Pokallus

Mental health stigma has been around for many generations. It is just recently that mental health is being prioritized by our society and treating mental health has become more and more popular. Mental health is defined as the emotional and psychological well-being of a person. It is very important to prioritize mental health in your everyday life for many reasons. Our emotional well-being affects our everyday lives, how well we perform in work settings, how we connect with friends and family, how we process and handle stress in our lives, and how we feel about ourselves in every stage of life.

Historically, mental health issues were linked to demons and spiritual possession which led to discrimination against those who suffered. These misguided views have led to centuries of stigma around mental health and mental health treatment. As the years went on, the belief that mental health issues were linked to possession faded away, but the stigma surrounding mental health did not.

Destigmatizing mental health is difficult with the years of internalizing that seeking help signifies weakness. This stigma may lead to reluctance to seek professional help, being misunderstood by family and peers, fewer career opportunities, harassment from others, social isolation, higher expenses due to little to no health insurance coverage for care, and the belief that there will be no improvement in emotional well-being.

In order to reduce the stigma around mental health treatment while also increasing the number of people exploring treatment, we need to speak openly about mental health issues and mental health treatment. We must first understand that there is nothing wrong with seeking mental help.

Everyone experiences stress related to work, family, or other personal situations, but for those who struggle with their mental health, this stress could impact them further. Just because others can handle the same or greater amounts of stress without seeking help, does not mean that personal struggles are not highly distressing. There is not one person on earth that shares the same background and personal struggles as anyone else; basing mental health barriers around others' lives is not sustainable.

The first way to destigmatize mental health is to seek treatment and be open and honest about it. The more people who talk about their struggles and how they coped, the more individuals not getting help will see that it is not as bad as perceived. Never let stigma create shame around seeking treatment, this could only cause self-doubt and uncertainty. Isolation is another factor that could cause problems; do not isolate yourself from those in your life. Your friends and family are important, isolation could only cause further mental health issues. Mental illness should never be factored into the evaluation of self-worth, this belief that individuals are only their illness further stigmatizes mental health and causes more problems for those suffering. Lastly, utilize the resources provided. Whether this is at school, from friends and family, or a support group, it is key to speak openly in a safe space about past and present struggles.

The stigma surrounding mental health has caused many issues for those who struggle with their mental health. It causes those who are already experiencing internal battles to also experience external battles. There is no positive to mental health stigma, it serves no purpose but to shame individuals. Even if you personally are not struggling, it is important to speak out about mental health stigma and help those around you.

Mental Health: The Reality of Getting Help

by Alix Greenblatt

Even with insurance, you may not receive the best service. While the concept of telehealth has become a revolutionary change for people seeking medical attention, not all services work that way, and one may have to find whatever is nearby. There have been stories about people, especially young ones, who seek services and feel like they left worse than when they came in. Misdiagnoses often lead to improper medication treatment and possible harm to the individual. The truth is the best insurance provides the best services, but the best insurance, consequently, costs more. Therefore, the more money one has, the more services they will be provided.

Everything mentioned is what occurs in the United States. In Europe, countries cover these types of services with free healthcare, making it easier for their citizens to receive help. The top nations with the top mental health services are Sweden, Germany, and Finland. The United States was ranked 3rd for the burden of mental health and doesn't even make the Top 20 in mental health services.

So, one question remains. Why does a country like the United States with one of the top economies in the world struggle so much to provide services for mental health? Stigma is always to blame. Mental health and mental healthcare have always been controversial discussions for nations around the world and it still is. In this country, the government and the people are divided. Traditional or conservative thinking on mental health has never been a pretty picture to paint, and you can see that with all the abandoned psychiatric centers that plague the country. You see it in Hollywood movies in the way they mock mental health, glamorize the struggle, and just flat-out get the idea wrong.

This all being said, many people–people in charge–do not want to fund services for mental health. It's a discussion that people want to keep hidden, hidden from those who need it most. People with money and power will always get the services they need. Just because one is more privileged, does not mean they are exempt from things like mental health, but they are exempt from struggling to find the services or medications they need.

Children and Mental Health

by Alix Greenblatt

Introduction: What is Mental Health?

What is mental health? Defined by the World Health Organization (WHO), mental health (MH) is a state of mental well-being that enables people to cope with the stresses of life, realize their abilities, learn and work well, and contribute to their community (WHO, 2022). While mental health disorders are included in the discussion, mental health is something experienced by all on various levels. The determinants of mental health can come in multiple forms. Individual psychological/biological factors including emotional skills, substance use, and genetics, can all factor into a person's vulnerability to mental health problems. Exposure to unfavorable social, economic, environmental, and geopolitical circumstances (i.e., poverty, violence, inequality, and environmental deprivation) can increase the risk of experiencing mental health conditions (WHO, 2022).

Mental Health Care Accessibility in the United States:

People with mental health disorders remain disproportionately vulnerable to barriers to healthcare access. As with most healthcare services, mental health services can become unaffordable without some form of copay. As of 2022, the cost of a psychiatric visit without insurance can range from $150-200. The evaluation ranges even higher, possibly being $300-$500. The cost of mental health therapy can average from $65-$200 per session. Aside from these services, centers for rehabilitation and behavioral centers (especially for children/adolescents/teens) are rarely covered by health insurance or school systems – if applicable. These facilities can cost a person thousands, if not tens of thousands, of dollars annually, biannually, or even just monthly.

From 2008 to 2019, the number of people aged 18 and older with any mental health disorder/illness increased from 39.8 million to 51.5 million, a 30% increase (Modi et. al., 2022). The United States has been facing an ever-growing mental health crisis. From 2009 to 2019, the share of high school students who reported experiencing persistent feelings of sadness and/or hopelessness increased by 41% (Modi et. al., 2022). In October 2021, the American Academy of Pediatrics (AAP), the American Academy of Child and Adolescent Psychiatry (AACAP), and the Children's Hospital Association (CHA) declared child and adolescent mental health a national emergency (Modi et. al., 2022).

Children Aged 3-17:
Amongst some of the most vulnerable populations to poor mental health are children. A person's medical autonomy (physical and mental) is not granted in most states until they are 18 years old. Until they are of legal age to make their own decisions, the parents or legal guardians decide what services and care are given to their children. Various mental health disorders and illnesses begin developing around the age of fourteen and older (although some can also develop as young as 3 to 5 years of age). Mental disorders can affect children across a range of sociodemographic characteristics; however, prevalence can vary. Boys have had higher rates than girls of being diagnosed with ADHD, behavioral or conduct problems, ASF, Tourette syndrome, and rates of suicide (Bitsko, 2022). Young girls are estimated to have a higher rate of depression, suicidal ideation, and attempted suicide (Bitsko, 2022). The prevalence of many mental

disorders/indicators differs by race and ethnicity. Additionally, evidence has shown that racial bias can result in certain behaviors being misinterpreted as disruptive (especially amongst children in the Black community). Misdiagnoses and overdiagnoses are more likely to occur as well, masking other forms of mental distress (Bitsko, 2022).

The analogy of a child's mind being a sponge when pertaining to skills/talent can also apply to the future of their mental health. The social interactions that children experience not only define their public character but their inner one as well. The most influential social interactions a child can go through often come from parents/guardians, other family, friends, schools, and the community (Garcia-Carrion et. al., 2019). Looking at Vygostsky's (1978) theory of cognitive development, cognitive abilities are socially guided and constructed with culture as a servable mediator and human interaction in a social/cultural context enhances learning (Garcia-Carrion et. al., 2019).

A Closer Look at the United States Youth:

As of 2022 in the United States, roughly 20% of children aged 3 to 17 have a mental, emotional, developmental, or behavioral disorder. Post-2019, suicidal behaviors of high school students increased by more than 40%, most apparent during the height of the COVID-19 pandemic (Agency for Healthcare Research and Quality, 2022). Between 2008 to 2020, the rates of death from suicide among people aged twelve and over increased by 16% – from 14 per 100,000 population to 16.3 per 100,000; the overall suicide death rate from 2018 to 2020 decreased an overall 10% (AHRQ, 2022).

The rate of death by suicide increased by 2% for Hispanic youths and decreased by 13% among non-Hispanic White youths (AHRQ, 2022). From 2007 to 2017, the suicide death rate increased for Black youths from 2.6 per 100,000 to 4.8 per

100,000 population (AHRQ, 2022). In 2020, the 12th leading cause of death in the United States was suicide overall. Also, suicide was the second leading cause for children aged 10 to 14 years and the third leading cause of death for people aged 15 to 24 years. For children or teens who identify as a part of the LGBTQ+ community, the risk of suicidal ideation/behavior is higher (AHRQ, 2022).

Overall, the most diagnosed MH disorders among children ages 3 to 17 (2016-2019) were attention deficit disorder (approx. six million), anxiety (approx. 5.8 million), behavior problems, and depression
(approx. 2.7 million). For adolescents aged 12 to 17, depression becomes more concerning due to the possible experience of major depressive episodes. From 2018 to 2019, 15.1% of those aged 12 to 17 experienced major depressive episodes (AHRQ, 2022). From 2008 to 2019, the percentage of adolescents aged 12 to 17 with a major depressive episode (in the last 12 months who received treatment) for non-Hispanic White children increased from 43.1% to 50.3% – this rate decreased to 49.1% in 2020 (AHRQ, 2022). The rate for Hispanic adolescents was 37% in 2020 and approximately 35% for Black adolescents in 2019 (AHRQ, 2022).

Closer Look: The LGBTQ+ Community:
As reported by The Trevor Project (2023), within the past year, 41% of the young people in the LGBTQ+ community had considered attempting suicide. Comparatively, transgender and nonbinary young people reported lower rates of attempting suicide when living with people who respected their pronouns (The Trevor Project, 2023). Thirty-eight percent of the LGBTQ+ young people found their home to be supportive and 56% of the community who wanted to seek mental health care within the past year were not able to access it. It has been reported that 1 in 3 young people in the LGBTQ+ community said their mental health decreased due

to anti-LGBTQ+ policies and legislation (The Trevor Project, 2023). Around 2 in 3 people said that hearing about potential state and/or local laws banning people from discussing LGBTQ+ people at school negatively affected their mental health as well (The Trevor Project, 2023).

A reported 67% of LGBTQ+ individuals experienced anxiety, and 54% reported experiencing symptoms of depression (The Trevor Project, 2023). Despite symptoms of anxiety, depression, and the ideation of harmful and/or suicidal behaviors, the young people of the LGBTQ+ community struggle to gain access to mental health care. Overall, 81% of LGBTQ+ young people wanted mental health care and 56% of them were unable to get it (The Trevor Project, 2023).

Some of the cited reasoning for this included:
- "I was afraid to talk about my mental health concerns with someone else."
- "I did not want to have to get my parent's/caregiver's permission."
- "I was afraid I wouldn't be taken seriously."
- "I could not afford it."
- "I was afraid it wouldn't work."

Current Interventions in the United States:
- The Centers for Disease Control and Prevention (CDC) has been working toward the following to improve access to mental health care for children:
- Improving strategies to connect families to mental health care
- Understanding gaps in the mental health workforce that serve children
- Investigate how funding policies can affect mental health care
- Understanding social determinants of health makes accessing mental health care harder

Some interventions that have been recommended for increasing the mental health of children and adolescents included positive coping strategies (Theberath et. al., 2022). This includes but is not limited to, actively reducing stress, connecting with friends and family members, engaging in physical activities, limiting leisure screen time, and cognitive restructuring (Theberath et. al., 2022). Cognitive restructuring is defined as a technique used in cognitive therapy and cognitive behavior therapy to help the client identify his or her self-defeating beliefs or cognitive distortions, refute them, and then modify them so that they are adaptive and reasonable (American Psychological Association, 2023). Schools and other community groups that children benefit from are crucial for keeping children and adolescents safe. These outlets assist them with finding proper mental health services when needed (Abrams, 2023). However, the COVID-19 pandemic disrupted these means of support due to constant isolation and online learning (Abrams, 2023). Abrams (2023) states that, from the perspective of health experts, the shortage of providers that are trained to meet the needs of children and adolescents is the biggest challenge faced for mental healthcare. Through the CDC programs for schools, they work to fund districts to update and improve classroom management, help implement service-learning programs for students, bring in mentors from the community into schools, and make the overall school system a safer, more supportive place for LGBTQ+ students. Prior to the COVID-19 Pandemic, the CDC found that girls, LGBTQ+ youth, and those who have experienced racism/bigotry were more likely to have poor mental health (Abrams, 2023). Some contributing factors were likely to include stigma, discrimination, and online bullying; concepts that were not foreign to pre-pandemic society (Abrams, 2023). The constant drive that young people have to seek approval from their peers, families, and other older individuals has also led to poor mental health outcomes, popularly seen from social media outlets. The unrealistic standards that society has set for people, especially young girls on their appearance, have led to further negative effects on one's mental health (Abrams, 2023).

Programs to train teachers and other school staff to create supportive classrooms while also aiding students who are in distress are currently being built by psychologists (Abrams, 2023). Developed by the Mental Health Technology Transfer Center Network and the University of Maryland's National Center for School Mental Health (NCSMH), Classroom WISE (Well-Being Information and Strategies for Educators) is an online course and resource library that draws on psychological research based around social-emotional learning, behavioral regulation, mental health literacy, trauma, and more (Abrams, 2023).

In addition to improving school systems, the expansion of the mental healthcare workforce is imperative to seeking better mental health for children and adolescents. Better screening and prevention measures, especially to decrease the need for intensive care, are included in this goal (Abrams, 2023). Established in 2006, New York launched a state-funded program, "The Ideas Center," for evidence-based treatment dissemination. The center offers free training on evidence-based practices for trauma, behavioral and attention problems, anxiety, depression, and more to all mental health professionals who work with children in the New York State licensed programs (Abrams, 2023). This includes but is not limited to, foster care, juvenile justice, and school settings (Abrams, 2023).

Conclusion:
The topic of mental health in the United States has been one that remains overlooked today. Mental health affects people of all ages and backgrounds, especially children and adolescents. This feature only touches the surface of the urgency surrounding mental health amongst young people, as well as interventions in the United States. This topic has been defined as a national emergency and should be treated as such. Young people need to feel supported and safe when it comes to their mental health, and this can start with education and the reduction of stigma. *Children are the future of this country and the world, and without proper mental healthcare, the future may look formidable.*

Relationships: Make or Break Work-Life Balance

by Kealan Connors

Work-life balance has been a topic for the last three years. Due to Covid-19, research has come out saying that relationships are the key to finding the right balance between work and life. These relationships can be in the form of friends, family, coworkers, and even their place of work. With these relationships, our need to thrive and better increases, and people generally have a more positive outlook on a situation.

This article will focus on four main points. The first one will be how weak-tie relationships relate to work-life balance. The proceeding point will be how weak-tie relationships lead to a lower burnout rate in nurses, and the next point will demonstrate how strong-tie relationships, such as living with a spouse and/or child, can lower depression scores. The last point will showcase how weak-tie relationships among management can create a better work-life balance for employees. These elements culminate into the main idea that relationships can either make or break work-life balance during the Covid-19 pandemic.

Weak-tie relationships and how they relate to work-life balance

Research into how weak-strong-tie relationships affect work-life balance found that weak-tie relationships offered better social support than strong-tie relationships. Weak-tie relationships, such as coworkers, acquaintances, and relative strangers, give individuals advice unheard of in strong-tie relationships with family members and friends. In an interview with Dr. Wright, he stated that the principle of homophily is the reason for higher support for weak-tie relationships. Dr. Wright noted that "people are more likely to bond with others who are similar to themselves. This similarity leaves space for differences of opinion and diverse responses to a situation. Weak-tie relationships offer opinions different from their own and allow people to process obstacles differently."

Dr. Wright explained, "Venting to a person not considered a close relationship allows for a safe communication climate and the ability to let off steam without worrying about hurting a family/friend's feelings." This allowed individuals to finally express themselves and feel less isolated and lonely.

Weak-tie support lead to a lower burnout rate

Weak-tie support also lowered the burnout rate for individuals working in a challenging job; according to Dr. Hocevar, "having colleagues who are going through the same struggles allows for a unique perspective that makes an individual continue to keep their head up and power through the struggles because they know that they are not alone. Family members can similarly support them, but coworkers offer a perspective only nurses can understand for careers in nursing and dealing with Covid in the hospitals." Weak-tie relationships offer the ability to calm work-life balance by being open-minded and offering ideas to power through the struggles of working from home.

Living with a partner and child increases a better work-life balance

Because of Covid-19, many families were forced to spend every hour of every day together. This could be either positive or negative. Dr. Wright and fellow researchers found that living with a spouse and a child had an overall increase in lowering depression scores. Dr. Wright believes this is due to the improved quality of time with their children. Before Covid, individuals had to drop their children off at school, clean the house, cook dinner, and spend most of their time at work. Now, with the children at home, these individuals can spend much more time with their spouses and children doing their favorite activities.

These strong ties cause depression, social isolation, and loneliness to drop dramatically. Others living alone do not have the same excuse to separate themselves from work. They spend even more time working than usual because they do not need to entertain anyone else. This strong-tie relationship shows their actual value. Forcing someone off the computer and becoming active with their friends and families allows for increased social engagement and a more positive outlook on their work-life balance.

A positive relationship with management makes for a better work-life balance

To create an outstanding work-life balance, employees must work with management. The relationship with management can allow the company to grow from a business to a weak-tie relationship with employees. Dr. Wright said, "By offering telecommunications, people do not have to travel as much. This allows people to be more productive and engaged in assignments." Businesses are a massive part of the everyday life of individuals. By creating opportunities for their employees, the burnout rate can drop, and the feeling of social isolation will ebb.

How do they all relate?

Weak and strong-tie relationships make work-life balance more fluid. People engaging in each other's situations by talking and understanding leads to a feeling of trust and security that makes work-life balance manageable. Businesses are built upon the relationships forged by weak and strong ties. They set themselves up as a successful business by engaging with employees and creating an open-door policy. In general, relationships are what make or break the work-life balance.

The Effects of Eating Disorders
by Courtney Pokallus

Eating disorders are one of the deadliest mental illnesses. There are multiple types of eating disorders including anorexia nervosa, bulimia nervosa, binge-eating disorder, and avoidant restrictive food intake disorder. Anorexia nervosa is the most fatal of the eating disorders with an extremely high mortality rate compared to other mental health disorders. Anorexia nervosa includes a restrictive subtype and a binge-purge subtype. Those with anorexia nervosa have a distorted body image, which is what causes them to restrict or binge and purge. Bulimia nervosa includes binge-eating, but also dispelling of the food to compensate for the binging. This disorder is also paired with a distorted body image like anorexia nervosa. Binge-eating disorder is different from bulimia nervosa as periods of binging are not followed by compensation, those who suffer from binge-eating also do not possess a distorted body image. Avoidant restrictive food intake disorder occurs when individuals limit the amount of food intake they consume, this is similar to anorexia nervosa except not as extreme and not paired with body image issues.

Eating disorders can affect anyone of any culture, background, size, and shape. They typically appear during teenage years and affect the individual into adulthood but can also occur later on in life. The effects of eating disorders on the human body are severe and can become irreversible. Eating disorders can lead to a number of health problems including heart problems, malnutrition, dehydration, slowed brain function, and gastrointestinal problems that can become permanent like bacterial infections, blood sugar fluctuations, nausea, stomach pain, bloating, and blocked intestines. Eating disorders can also cause a decrease in hormone levels, hypothermia, and deterioration of the esophagus as well as teeth, and in severe cases, they can lead to death.

Coming in at the second highest mortality rate of all mental illnesses behind opioid misuse disorder, an individual dies every fifty-two minutes as a direct result of an eating disorder. Those who suffer from eating disorders are more likely to die prematurely due to inadequate nutrition, but they are also more likely to become addicted to drugs which also could lead to their death. Eating disorders also deteriorate the quality of life for those affected. When suffering from an eating disorder, individuals tend to only think about their food intake and calorie count, and stress about how these things could affect their body.

Treating eating disorders as early as possible is crucial to help the individual get back on track. There are multiple forms of treatments for eating disorders depending on severity and preference; this includes individual or group psychotherapies which include help from families to feed the individual more or cognitive behavioral therapies to help the individual identify their habits and behaviors. Medications such as antipsychotics, antidepressants, and mood stabilizers are utilized to treat eating disorders and other mental health problems that could coincide, like anxiety and depression. There is also nutritional counseling and medical monitoring of patients to improve nutritional habits.

Eating disorders are life-threatening mental disorders that greatly impact an individual's life. It is important to understand the signs and symptoms of someone with an eating disorder in order to identify destructive habits as early as possible. Some symptoms of eating disorders include extremely restrictive eating, as well as extreme thinness or looking emaciated, fear of gaining weight and body image issues, brittle hair and nails, osteoporosis or osteopenia, acid reflux disorder, intestinal distress, eating an unusual amount of food or eating when not hungry, guilt about food intake, dramatic weight loss or weight gain, and frequent dieting. It is crucial to identify the signs of eating disorders to aid the individual in receiving treatment, as waiting could result in irreversible damage to many organs or even death.

Attention Deficit Hyperactivity Disorder Connected with Depression

By Anooshka Shukla

Mental Health Impact Within Public Health

Recently, there has been a surge concerning how mental health impacts the overall score of global public health. The World Health Organization (2022) states that within the last decade, mental health and substance use conditions have risen to 13%. Additionally, mental health costs one trillion dollars to the global economy (WHO, 2022). There have been various mental health conditions that persistently cause distress and disruption in daily life, routine, and activity, such as depression, anxiety, attention deficit disorder, and schizophrenia. There have also been a variety of mental health organizations that focus on assisting people afflicted with mental health conditions and educating the public about symptoms of mental distress and health conditions.

Depression

Depression is a mental health condition characterized by symptoms such as guilt, sadness, and worthlessness (Healthline, 2016). Depression is cited as one of the most common mental health conditions with 5% of adults suffering from depression globally (WHO, 2022). Depression usually exists either as a singular health condition or as an additional condition (co-morbidity) to another health condition. One example to note is depression existing with heart failure. Sbolli et al. (2020) examine the connection between depression and heart failure, stating that depression greatly affects heart failure patients through worse quality-of-life conditions and outcomes. Depression can affect anyone in any demographic, which is the reason for many campaigns not only calling awareness for the symptoms of this mental health issue but also various resources to combat its symptoms. Some resources can be found online to treat depression via a holistic-medical approach, as well as ad campaigns that spread awareness about the debilitating effects of depression and the understanding of a daily routine under depression.

Attention Deficit Hyperactivity Disorder

Attention Deficit Hyperactivity Disorder, also known as ADHD, is a mental health issue that is characterized by symptoms of struggling in focus, self-control, and restlessness (NIMH, n.d.). Attention Deficit Hyperactivity Disorder has been mostly known as a mental health issue that occurs during childhood and adolescence. However, it can persist through adulthood, with the overall prevalence of adult ADHD is 4.4% (NIMH, n.d.). ADHD also has the potential for co-morbidities, such as anxiety and conduct disorder (Magnus et al., 2022). However, it is also stated to be easily treatable with properly prescribed medications (Magnus et al., 2022).

The Connection Between Depression and ADHD

There are studies that research the causal relationship between depression and attention deficit hyperactivity disorder. Powell et al. (2021) state individuals affected with ADHD would be at more risk of depression. Additionally, they found that out of 148 participants, 12.4% who had depression also had ADHD symptoms and 3.4% met the criteria for ADHD (Powell et al., 2021). What this signifies is that those who are afflicted with depression, particularly recurrent depression, are also viable for exhibiting symptoms of ADHD. Another study also touched upon this relationship between depression and attention deficit hyperactivity disorder (ADHD). Riglin et al. (2021) state that there is considerable genetic overlap between ADHD and depression. It is further explained that their MR analyses suggest a causal relationship of ADHD genetic liability regarding depression (Riglin et al., 2021). What this signifies is that there is a genetic reason why depression and ADHD are comorbidities with each other. While it might not always result in both mental health issues existing together always, there is a strong relationship regarding the genetic disposition for both ADHD and depression linking them together.

Conclusion:
With mental health becoming an integral part of public health, many research studies focus on comorbidities regarding mental health conditions. Depression is linked to Attention Deficit Hyperactivity Disorder (ADHD) through genetic overlap, which makes their comorbidity just as likely to occur as depression-anxiety comorbidity. However, as research into this relationship progresses, so does the underlying complexity of tackling this type of mental health dilemma.

Mental Health in Minority Group Communities

by Alix Greenblatt

Amongst many of the important topics throughout the month of July is National Minority Mental Health Awareness. Each July, this topic is observed to bring awareness to the struggle that racial and ethnic minority communities face within the United States. People from these communities often suffer from lower/poor mental health due to high rates of inaccessibility to high quality mental health services, cultural stigmas that surround the topic of mental health, discrimination, and a lack of awareness.

General Information

According to the Mental Health in America Report (2023), 21% of adults in the United States are experiencing mental health disorders or illness- equivalent to 50 million Americans. Around 55% of adults with a mental illness receive no treatment- equivalent to 28 million people. Over 5.5 million adults (11%) with a mental illness are uninsured and 28% of adults with a mental illness reported that they are not able to receive the treatments they need. The report will be provided below.

Minority Implications

People from minority group communities are more likely to experience discrimination in the healthcare community, with a high possibility of not being able to receive health insurance. Around ⅓ or 33% of the United States population are without some form of health insurance. As of 2021, uninsured groups in the United States ranged from 5.7% (White), 10.9% (Black) 18.8% (non-Hispanic identifying as American Indian/Alaska

Native), and 17.7% (Hispanic or Latino). Without health insurance, the access to mental health services (i.e., psychiatry, mental health therapy, rehabilitation centers) tremendously decreases.

Issues Attaining Mental Health Care

As with most healthcare services, mental health services can become unaffordable without some form of co-pay. As of 2022, the cost of a psychiatric visit without insurance can range from $150-200. The evaluation ranges even higher, possibly being $300-$500. The cost of mental health therapy can average from $65-$200 per session. Aside from these services, centers for rehabilitation and behavioral centers (especially for children/adolescents/teens) are rarely covered by health insurances or school systems- if applicable. These facilities can cost a person thousands, if not tens of thousands of dollars annually, biannually, or even just monthly.

While these concerns do not reach those of a higher economic status, the reality is that many people do have this concern and there is little action being taken. As of this year, the current U.S. administration has stated they would take action to tackle the nation's Mental Health Crisis. Some actions include funding $200 million to scale up around 988 suicide/crisis lifelines and provide new resources for school-based mental health services. The administration has made a plan to increase the size and diversity of the behavioral health workforce, expand access to peer support, enhance the crisis response, and to make it easier to seek help.

The Chronically Ill

Advocating for those with chronic illness is another major priority for our public health system. Unfortunately, there is an increasing amount of patients who face the physical pain, the emotional pain, and the financial burdens of living with a chronic disease. However, the bright side of the situation is that our public health system is always working with medical centers throughout the country as well as the Food and Drug Administration to find new options for making the symptoms of chronic disease more manageable. At the same time, the public health system provides extensive current updates and education for chronically ill patients, to help them cope with their diseases, as well as programs that offer assistance for emotional counselling and financial help. In addition, many patients with chronic disease need the help of caregivers. The public health system needs to intensify its programs and support for caregivers, as well. Perhaps one of the most devastating diseases facing many Americans and their families is Alzheimer's Disease. The commentary that follows provides an overview of the life of a caregiver.

- Bob Kieserman

How to Support Someone with Alzheimer's

by Faalik Zahra

Do you have a loved one that has Alzheimer's? You are not alone. In 2022, there was an estimated 6 million people who have Alzheimer's in America. It is difficult to see a loved one experience so much because of the disease's impact. People in the patient's support group often feel helpless.

First, it is essential to understand what Alzheimer's disease is. The Alzheimer's Association, a voluntary health organization, describes Alzheimer's as "the most common cause of dementia, a general term for memory loss and other cognitive abilities serious enough to interfere with daily life." Some symptoms that the individual may experience are memory loss, confusion, social withdrawal, and difficulty completing tasks. The symptoms may be at different levels depending on the individual.

Understanding Alzheimer's and its impact will assist you in understanding how you can help. Individuals often need help with tasks throughout their day and assistance in alleviating their confusion. For this, they need to have a support system to aid them.

Motivating the individual to perform different tasks and partake in activities is essential. Many patients often remove themselves from work and social activities, which can impact their mental health. Incorporating a routine in the individual's life can help ensure this doesn't happen. What works best for an individual differs from person to person, but small activities, social interactions, and routines can help the caregiver decide what works best.

Throughout this process, as a caregiver, it is important to take care of yourself as well. It is a challenging and stressful time for the family and loved ones of patients with Alzheimer's. It is essential for you to take care of yourself, ask for help, and join a support group. It is important to remember that if you don't take care of yourself, you will not be able to take care of others.

If you do not know someone directly impacted by Alzheimer's, you can still help! You can create awareness of Alzheimer's and educate others around you. November is Alzheimer's Awareness month, making it a great way to get involved and impact. Professionals are continuously researching Alzheimer's treatment options and donating to fund these projects can go a long way. These projects focus on combating Alzheimer's and finding preventative measures that can help diminish its impact. Together we can help fight Alzheimer's.

Safe Neighborhoods

The public health system advocates for safer neighborhoods because when people live without fear, their overall health is improved. Without fear, people are not afraid to go to a doctor's office or a clinic for medical care, and they are not fearful of walking or travelling to a pharmacy to get needed medicine. We live in a society plagued with a lack of gun control, which leads to senseless violence, and in too many neighborhoods, inadequate and unsafe housing and poverty. To improve this situation, public health advocates work endlessly to create and implement programs that focus on building communities, eliminating domestic violence and street violence, improving the safety of public transportation, making pharmacies and healthcare facilities more accessible to communities, and educating residents on better and safer housing options. The public heath advocates also focus on creating and implementing programs that provide employment opportunities that lead to self-respect and self-reliance.

- Bob Kieserman

Advocating for Safe Neighborhoods

by Caitlin Laska

The idea of neighborhoods and housing as social determinants of health is a newer concept. In the past, health focused on individual characteristics such as behaviors, psychological traits, biological predispositions, and social class. At the time, there was little focus on other factors in the community and neighborhood. However, the study of communities and neighborhoods as a social determinant of health has significantly grown and impacted how public health approaches inequalities.

How do we define a neighborhood in public health?
Neighborhoods are the environment in which we live, work, and grow. This encompasses daily exposures, like pollution, the physical environment, such as distance from green spaces, and the social environment, namely violence. Neighborhoods also bring together several social determinants of health, including socioeconomic status, access to food, and race. Let's look at the example of a person who lives near a park and has access to a grocery store with fresh fruits and vegetables in a neighborhood with low crime. This person can easily be physically active by going for a walk in the park. They can also access fresh foods that will help prevent obesity, diabetes, and heart disease. Finally, they will feel safe coming home late from work, which will reduce stress. On the other hand, a person who lives near a highway, across the street from a convenience store, and in a high-crime area would live a completely different life. They could have asthma from the air pollution caused by living next to a highway. In addition, the convenience store likely sells tobacco and alcohol, which can increase the person's likelihood of drinking and smoking. Finally, they would face psychological stressors from violence

in the community. As these examples illustrate, neighborhoods impact us socially and physically, and the more we understand about this, the better we can make our communities.

Pollution

Pollution is a major contributor to the quality of life. Examples include but are not limited to, air pollution, smoke, chemicals (such as lead and hazardous waste), and water quality. Air pollution and smoke have been shown to cause asthma. According to the Cleveland Clinic, smoking irritates the moist lining of the lungs and damages cilia which help sweep dust and mucus out of the lungs. Second-hand smoke, which includes tar, carbon monoxide, and nicotine, is just as harmful. Children are especially at risk of developing respiratory diseases since their lungs are smaller and still maturing. Exposure to smoke inflames the airways and children with asthma are especially sensitive. They are more likely to develop lung and sinus infections and have worse asthma attacks. Smoking or living with a smoker can severely impact one's health and those around them. High levels of pollution have the same effect. Neighborhoods near a highway, factory, or airport tend to have increased levels of air pollution and, therefore, more asthma cases.

Another example of pollution is chemical toxins found around the house. Examples include lead from lead paint and asbestos. These toxins are common in older houses and apartments and must be checked to ensure they are safe. The National Cancer Institute says that prolonged asbestos exposure can cause cancer such as mesothelioma, lung, larynx, and ovarian cancer. On the other hand, according to the CDC, lead exposure causes brain and nervous system damage, slowed development, learning and behavior problems, and hearing and speech problems. Lead poisoning is most common in children. As children learn to crawl and explore, they may accidentally ingest lead paint chips or dust. Lead contamination is also a problem in water pipes and may not be detected until symptoms have already begun.

Water contamination is another form of pollution that still plagues America. In 2014, the country saw the horrid effects of polluted water in Flint, Michigan. A combination of lead pipes and Legionella bacteria created a major disaster in the region, whose full effects will not be known for years to come. There are currently 12 deaths and 90 illnesses linked back to the contaminated water. Access to clean drinking water is vital for a healthy neighborhood. Citizens need to trust that their water is safe from chemical and biological contaminants, and it is the city's job to ensure this. In areas that lack funding, as seen with Flint, pipes may not be changed or regulated. This can result in catastrophic consequences and shows how clean drinking water impacts the quality of a neighborhood and its health.

Physical Environment
The physical environment of a neighborhood encompasses location and quality of housing. The location where one lives significantly impacts health. For example, proximity to grocery stores plays a major role in what the community eats. Grocery stores dictate what type and quality of food the community has access to. If there are no fresh foods like fruits and vegetables nearby, a community may see higher rates of obesity, diabetes, and heart disease. In addition, proximity to convenience stores where tobacco and alcohol are sold influences the number of people who smoke and drink. A National Health Institute article found that there is a positive association between tobacco retail store density and smoking behaviors, especially among youth. Finally, according to the CDC, proximity to bike lanes, sidewalks, and green spaces

dictate how likely a person is to go outside to exercise. People who have more access to parks and trails tend to be more physically active. However, less than half of Americans live within a half mile of a park.

The quality of one's housing can also predict their health status. According to Healthy People 2030, a report from the Department of Health and Human Services, a lack of air conditioning and heating has been correlated with high blood pressure, respiratory illness, and depression. For many, air conditioning is a luxury and too expensive to install, and both AC and heating are costly to run. Further, water leaks that go untreated can cause mold growth leading to respiratory infections, asthma, and coughing. Oftentimes mold is not visible and may not be found until symptoms have arisen. Finally, the lack of smoke alarms and carbon monoxide detectors can lead to injury and death. According to the U.S. Consumer Product Safety Commission, three-out-of five deaths from house fires occurred in homes without working smoke alarms. Oftentimes, low-income communities take the brunt of these issues.
Ensuring home safety is vital for a healthy neighborhood.

Social Environment
The social environment of a neighborhood encompasses how the residents feel in the neighborhood. Is it a safe area? Is there drug use? Safety features, such as crime rates and drug use, severely impact the neighborhood's health. In fact, the U.S. Department of Justice considers exposure to violence a "national crisis" that must be addressed and further studied. A study published in the American Journal of Psychology studied the correlation between mental health and areas of crime. It found that rates of PTSD are 85% higher in high-crime rate areas compared to low-crime rate areas. Further,

the study noted that 14.8% of residents in areas with violent crime met the diagnosis of depression. In addition, crime disrupts sleep and cortisol (stress hormone) levels. A study from Northwestern University found that the day after a crime, residents went to bed two hours later and woke up with higher levels of cortisol. While waking up feeling stressed is a part of life, continuous stress from living in a violent area has been shown to lower academic performance. No matter the age, residents in crime-ridden areas are at a disadvantage.

Drug use is also an indicator of a neighborhood's health. A study published in the American Journal of Health Behavior found that perceived fear of the neighborhood's environment is positively associated with drug use. While everyone experiences some level of stress, the American Psychological Association says that repeated exposure to stress is thought to increase the risk of hypertension, heart attack, and stroke. Residents should feel safe to leave their homes and go outside, and drug use takes away from this. As these examples show, crime and drug use significantly impact a community's mental health.

Provider Burnout

In recent years, large for-profit corporations and large hospital systems have changed the landscape of healthcare delivery. As a result, many older and experienced physicians and other healthcare providers have retired or left medicine to pursue other careers because of the stress of working for these organizations. As one older doctor was quick to say, "I am not practicing the medicine that I once practiced. Today, the focus is no longer on patient centered care, but rather improving the bottom line. Where before I could take my time with a patient and give them my full attention with a complete examination, now I am limited to 10 minutes, and spend most of the time looking at the computer, rather than sitting down with my patient".

As a result, two things have occurred affecting our public health system. One is that many providers have experienced burnout to the extent that some will admit that they can no longer provide quality care, and the other is that with the retirement of many providers, who have been caring for their patients for decades, it has left many patients with the need to find new doctors, and many of these patients are elderly, and the change is difficult. At the same time, the shortage of nurses, which has been going on for years now, is also becoming a public health crisis, since patients are dependent on nurses to care for them in the hospital as well as at home.

In a 2023 statement by the American Medical Association, it was reported that the highest percentages of burnout occurred in six medical specialties: emergency medicine (62%), hospital medicine (59%), family medicine (58%), pediatrics (55%), OB/GYN (54%) and internal medicine (52%). Clearly, this indicates a shortage of doctors who we depend upon to handle our emergency care, who oversee our care when we are hospitalized, our primary care, the care of our children, care for women who are pregnant, and the care of the elderly. To patients throughout the country, this is indeed a public health crisis.

This next section discusses this public health issue and its important ramifications.

- Bob Kieserman

Physician Burnout

by Maia Signore

When walking into a doctor's office, patients' main concern is their well-being; they don't necessarily think about how their physician is doing or if they are okay. Many times, physicians have the same issues their own patients have, but they can't show it while at work. Physician burnout is a prolonged response due to chronic occupational stressors.

Symptoms of physician burnout include but are not limited to, high levels of exhaustion, which is caused by working long hours, as well as limited breaks due to unpredictable circumstances. Depression is also a major symptom, which is caused by not being home because of long hours, not seeing their family and friends enough, and the same routine every day that eventually becomes old and "lifeless." Finally, there is a lack of efficacy caused by a lack of motivation to keep going after so many negative results in patients. What also contributes to the lack of efficacy is the lack of time that is spent outside the workplace, because even when physicians are home, a lot of the time, they are still working.

As we know, with symptoms come causes. Many factors result in physician burnout including poor work and life balance, loss of autonomy, decreased control over the work environment, poor management in the healthcare setting, and COVID-19 playing a major role. Physicians are spending so much time at the workplace that they don't get to have the social life they sometimes desire or the family time they need; therefore, they are left feeling like they live at work. Physicians are also required to use specific practices at their workplace which can overall lead to health disparities or worse. This often makes physicians feel a need to seek out different workplaces or additional resources. Physicians are losing a sense of control when practicing their own medicine due to surrounding factors like administration, ever-changing policies/rules, as well as standards they are set to. These are examples of how loss of autonomy and decreased control over the work environment have contributed to physician burnout. Lastly, COVID-19 became a major factor in physician burnout. The ongoing pandemic created even longer working hours, unsafe working conditions, and high levels of stress that physicians are still experiencing today.

How does physician burnout affect patients? There is less time spent with the patients, so appointments that used to be 20-30 minutes long are now 10-15 minutes, at times due to the overload of scheduling for doctors. This leads to a decreased quality of care, meaning patient's symptoms/concerns are often overlooked and not taken into consideration which can result in medical error. As a result, high medical error has become an additional contributor to the effects of physician burnout. This can result in the wrong medication prescribed, the wrong diagnosis, and even patients being told nothing is wrong.

So how can we help reduce physician burnout? Teamwork is a big factor that can help, as well as acknowledgment of hard work, working together in treating patients, and side work can significantly help in treating physician burnout because it takes some of the stress and work off the individual physicians. Additionally, reducing the number of tasks physicians have to do that do not involve patient care would make it so that physicians are focusing more on their patients and themselves. With symptoms of depression comes time and space to help them mentally and physically. Giving physicians time off when necessary and allowing flexibility can help doctors' mental health as well, which is extremely important for everyone especially doctors when they are treating patients for their own illnesses. This leads to the point of creating a healthy environment by providing mental health support and wellness programs as part of the workplace. If our physicians aren't doing well mentally, that will be taken out on the patients as well as co-workers. Finally, address burnout in training and/or in the early stages so that it is caught and resolved before it worsens to the point of no return.

In conclusion, in order for our patients to be happy and healthy, our physicians need to be also. The examples mentioned prior are just a small part of what to look for in physicians regarding burnout, and the solutions/treatment options can help physicians immensely.

Physician Burnout: The Crisis and Possible Resolutions
by Emma Nolan

What is the issue of physician burnout? Burnout can be described as, "a psychological syndrome emerging as a prolonged response to chronic interpersonal stressors on the job". The term was originally coined by clinical psychologist Herbert Freudenberger in 1974 who spoke of burnout as exhaustion that occurred among "the dedicated and the committed". It has been more recently characterized by cynical or negative attitudes towards patients, emotional exhaustion, feelings of decreased personal achievement, and lack of empathy for patients.

Burnout is heavily affecting physicians, with 46% of physicians reporting burnout in 2015 and the numbers continuing on an upwards trend. Having a higher degree typically decreases the chances of burnout occurring, but when that degree is a M.D. or D.O., the chances of burnout actually increase. So what exactly is causing these high levels of burnout in this field? The answer is a combination of factors ranging from stress to poor work/life balance to flaws in the healthcare system itself.

Possible Reasons: Longer Hours, Government Regulations, and Stress
Working long hours may come naturally to physicians, seeing as their goal is to help people and more often than not, put others' needs ahead of their own. This may mean staying late in the office with patients, filling out paperwork, or getting ready for the next day. These long hours combined with the stressors of the career do not

mix well leading to this feeling of burnout. The way in which the healthcare system is set up also tends to lead to physician burnout. Pressures from the management of the hospital or the office practice to see as many patients as possible can lead to decreased time spent with patients. In 2009, the Health Information Technology for Economic and Clinical Health (HITECH) Act was passed which had most hospitals in the country switch to Electronic Health Records (EHRs). The United States provided monetary incentives for those who did so and imposed Medicare and Medicaid reimbursement restrictions to those who did not. Even though this act brought about many changes that were needed, it led to some physicians feeling overwhelmed. New regulations were brought about that aimed to enhance practice efficiency, meaning a higher amount of patients must be seen in a day. This led to shortened visit times and less time understanding and connecting with the patients. Even though HITECH has numerous benefits in healthcare, more efficiency may not be what the physicians need.

Loss of Autonomy

Loss of autonomy is another huge factor contributing to high rates of physician burnout. Seeing higher amounts of patients plays a big role in loss of autonomy. In medicine, autonomy could mean deciding how much time the patient requires, what type of treatment they require, or when to schedule their next appointment. The policies that HITECH and other healthcare policies have put into place are the opposite of what physicians need in terms of greater autonomy. Higher turnover rates for rooms force the doctors to work on a time crunch and treat medicine as a so called "fixing-people production line". Researchers who focus on this topic have argued that doctors need time to be their patients to fully understand the reason for the visit, connect with them, and determine the best course of treatment.

The Pandemic Adds to the Pressures

The COVID-19 pandemic has continued to exacerbate physician burnout. Kaiser Family Foundation released the results from a recent poll that stated 6 in 10 health care workers have been dealing with mental health struggles since the start of the pandemic and half are feeling symptoms of burnout. The high number of cases of COVID-19 led to hospitals being overwhelmed with patients and not enough healthcare workers, and in some cases not enough beds and ventilators for the sick individuals. The main causes of increased levels of physician burnout since the start of the pandemic include treating patients who were likely to die, being exposed on a regular basis to COVID-19, and personal protective equipment not being readily available. Another study found more causes to include not having time with friends and family, lack of communication, and needing to take care of children who were doing virtual school. All of these stressors, on top of regular stressors of the career field, have exacerbated levels of physician burnout, not only in the U.S. but globally.

Possible Ways to Reduce Physician Burnout

Although we continue to see rising rates of physician burnout, there are measures being taken that aim to alleviate this current phenomenon. These measures are ranging from steps the physicians can take themselves to organizational interventions.

Physicians Becoming Proactive About Their Mental Health

The physicians themselves can help to combat burnout by recognizing the symptoms and being proactive. The Maslach Burnout Inventory (MBI) is commonly used to measure feelings of burnout. This questionnaire uses three measures which are: exhaustion, depersonalization, and personal accomplishment/efficacy. Although MBI is not a perfect tool, it does help with taking the steps to recognize the early symptoms of burnout. Just recognizing symptoms is not enough though. Physicians need to be able to take some time off and have ample access to mental health resources in order to reduce these feelings and learn ways to cope with work stressors. Health care organizations can also work towards supporting their doctors. The Charter for Physician Well Being was created by the Collaborative for Healing and Renewal in Medicine and aims to help promote physician well being. Goals for this charter include advocating for policies that benefit physician well being, building support systems within the organization, and creating a healthy work environment, among others. It is promising to see the current steps being taken to tackle this issue of physician burnout. But with the rising rates, especially since the start of the COVID-19 pandemic, additional steps must be implemented to protect the physicians that are working to keep the people of this country healthy.

How can patients help?
According to Bob Kieserman, Executive Director of The Power of the Patient Project: The National Library of Patient Rights and Advocacy and Project Director of MedFocus Research, its research division, patients can help reduce physician burnout by being more understanding and showing patience with their providers. As patients need their providers to be supportive, physicians need similar support from their patients. A simple gesture of asking a doctor how he or she is doing during a routine visit can sometimes open up a short conversation where the doctor will vent about some of the frustrations the doctor is feeling, and by the patient showing empathy, the stress felt by

the doctor can be reduced and a strong patient/provider connection can be achieved at the same time. Patients can also agree to have a medical scribe in the examination room to allow the doctor to have more face time with the patient and be less focused on a laptop to take notes throughout the visit, a need brought about by the electronic medical record system. In practices where medical scribes are not yet used, patients can also suggest to their doctor or the practice administrator that the use of medical scribes can be a help for the doctor. Finally, according to Kieserman, patients can talk to practice administrators and hospital administrators about how the patients feel about the patient encounter and whether the patient feels rushed through the visit, whether they feel their doctor is able to listen to them with full attention or not, and whether they feel that the method of scheduling patients is working. Patient feedback can be invaluable to making changes in the way the doctor is able to practice medical in both the office setting and the hospital setting. And perhaps, this can lessen the stress experienced by physicians and other healthcare providers.

The Nursing Shortage: What Patients Can Expect

By Cori Ritchey

"By the time I am done with my 12-hour shift, it feels like an eternity," a nurse reflects on her work. "The last thing you want to think about is having to return the next day and do it all again."

Alessia Smith is a registered nurse on a surgical and telemetry floor at a hospital outside of Boston. She is a recent graduate and has only been in the field for about seven months. To her, however, it "feels like a lifetime."

"Being understaffed affects everyone at work–the patients, the nurses, the secretary; sometimes, even the families of the patients we are taking care of," says Smith.

The nursing shortage is rattling hospitals, long-term facilities, and outpatient doctor's offices alike. The lack of workers creates a heavy burden on the few remaining, as patients pile up through the coronavirus pandemic, amongst other illnesses.

The factors that link to the current nursing shortage seem endless. On top of a worldwide pandemic that is building on already problematic burnout, there's already a whole generation of healthcare workers that are getting to the point of retirement.

"Baby boomers," those born between the years of 1946 and 1964, are currently hitting retirement age. According to a study done by the U.S. Department of Health and Human Services in 2018, 47.5 percent of RNs are over the age of 50.

Because of these new retirees, not only are we losing more and more nurses to retirement, but there is also an increasing number of senior citizens with aging bodies that need more healthcare. According to the National Library of Medicine, the 65+ population has increased by nearly 73 percent from 2011 to 2019, from 41 million to 71 million.

Some areas have been hit harder than others, regarding demographics. Texas, California, South Carolina, and Nevada have the worst nurse-to-population ratio. South Carolina ranks the lowest with only 7.9 registered nurses per 1000 people, according to a 2020 study from the University of Saint Augustine.

As the shortage continues, what can patients expect?

Patients should expect to be waiting a little longer for common needs, such as a pitcher of water or a blanket. The nurses that remain have to focus on prioritizing patient needs when there are fewer hands on deck.

"People are flooding the hospital with covid, and their symptoms are very crucial and sometimes we need to prioritize who we see first," Smith says. "My patients are very sick, and I tend to the ones that I feel need me the most."

Because of the lack of nurses, patients can also expect shortened lengths of stay. Doctors and hospital administrators will aim to discharge patients right when they are independent enough to be safe at home to relieve the ratio of patients to nurses.

Another thing patients need to expect is less small talk than normal.

"We aren't running out of [our patient's] room while they are mid-sentence telling us stories about their life or family just because we don't want to take the time to get to know them," Mary Zellhart, a registered nurse at the University of Vermont hospital, tells. "We are running because we heard someone yell for help from another room or a crisis 'high alert' alarm is going off which means a patient might be in critical condition and needs to be assessed quickly."

Patients will need to harness their patience through these times. They can help by keeping nurse calls to a minimum–asking for multiple things in one go rather than calling each time they need something.

"If [patients] can make a list of things they need the next time we come around to them for us to address instead of ringing multiple times in a short time span," Zellhart says. "This allows us to manage our time better and provide better quality of care."

The nurses who remain do their best to promptly accommodate patient needs and wants. Through this shortage, patients must respect longer wait times and prioritize what is important to ask for.

Patient Education and Health Literacy

One of the major roles of the public health system is to educate. Consequently, the most reliable information on medical advancements, new safety protocols like wearing a mask during the pandemic, advice on immunizations, teaching pregnant women how to better take care of themselves and their babies, and many more valuable lessons are shared with the American public every week by the public health system. People rely on these messages and updates to stay aware of any spread of disease, medicines and medical treatments that can help those who are ill, reminders about being screened for diseases like cancer and getting annual checkups, and what to expect from healthcare providers when a patient visits a doctor. Hundreds of hours are dedicated to educating all of us about what we need to know to stay healthier and safer, and we are fortunate that the public health system counts on the leading experts in the country to focus on patient education and making us all smarter consumers of healthcare. This next section provides insights on the depth of the patient education and health literacy initiatives of our public health system.

- Bob Kieserman

The Importance of Health Literacy
by Aidan Strealy

Every patient on earth has a body to take care of, and, therefore, every patient on earth can benefit from learning how to maintain it, adjust for chronic conditions, and handle the day-to-day affairs of sickness and injury. According to the American Academy of Family Physicians, the leading causes of death in the United States include heart disease, cancer, lung disease, and strokes. These conditions are often tied to unhealthy lifestyles, which can be improved by learning about the benefits of dieting, exercising regularly, and seeking care when ill. Through enhanced patient education, patients develop better health literacy that aids them in making more informed decisions about their bodies.

Health literacy is defined by the Health Resources and Services Administration as "the degree to which individuals have the ability to find, understand, and use information and services to inform health-related decisions and actions for themselves and others." While it might seem obvious to some, health literacy can be as simple as understanding a physician's instructions, following the directions on medication, or finding the right physician for their needs. When someone lacks health literacy, they may fail to take advantage of their resources, thereby becoming sicker. A study by Hickey et al. (2019) in the National Library of Medicine reports that patients who lack health literacy are hospitalized more often, develop more diseases, and have a higher rate of mortality than those with better health literacy.

Thankfully, these outcomes are not set in stone, as patient education and health literacy can be improved. One way of helping patients is by providing clear and accessible health information materials. Some clinics have brochures that outline different conditions or medications, which allows patients to revisit the most important topics discussed during an appointment. Another popular resource is the internet. Although there can be a lot of clutter to sort through, trusted websites like WebMD, the Mayo Clinic, and Healthline can provide valuable information within minutes. Having these resources available is crucial for healthcare entities and educative bodies because as with any type of learning, obstacles can get in the way.

One example of an obstacle is a language barrier. Although many Americans take it for granted that they can read, write, and speak the primary language of our healthcare system, there are plenty who cannot. If technical information about medications, treatments, or diagnoses is misunderstood, the patient will not be well-equipped to manage their condition. One way this has been addressed is by partnering with translator companies. For instance, Loma Linda University Hospital in Southern California has a welcome sign in over twenty different languages, explaining that if the patient does not feel confident conducting the visit in English, the hospital can call a translator to help things run more smoothly.

Another obstacle can lie in the cultural differences between a patient and their healthcare provider. If the patient follows a tradition placing less emphasis on Western Medicine, they might be less likely to engage with the American healthcare system, which, therefore, places greater importance on community organizations and other third-party groups working to improve health literacy. For example, the Society for Public Health Education (SOPHE) raises awareness about how to live healthier lives, whereas groups like the World Health Organization (WHO) operate on a larger scale to improve the health of entire nations. While they may vary in their methods, each of these organizations understands that improving patient education and health literacy will lead to a healthier world.

By empowering individuals with the knowledge and the understanding, patients will be better able to make informed decisions about their health and well-being. Effective patient education promotes better communication between healthcare providers and patients, leading to improved healthcare outcomes and enhanced patient satisfaction. Moreover, investing in health literacy initiatives will help eliminate the obstacles patients currently face, leading to a population better able to manage their health with fewer chronic conditions, and, therefore, fewer deaths nationwide.

The Importance of Patient Advocacy
by Maia Signore

Patient rights and advocacy are described as catering to a patient's unmet needs which includes informing, protecting, and speaking on behalf of patients, this is to ensure that patient rights are protected. There are three core values regarding patient advocacy: safeguarding patient autonomy, acting on behalf of patients, and promoting social justice in healthcare. Now patient advocacy radiates both positive and negative effects if correct, or not correct, measures are taken. Positive patient advocacy includes increased professional satisfaction, self-confidence, and self-esteem, as well as maintenance of personal integrity and moral principles. Negative consequences might include loss of reputation, friends, and self-esteem but can also lead to moral stress or dilemma. Physicians and staff have been let go of their jobs because of wrongdoing regarding patient rights and advocacy.

What does a patient advocate do?

Advocates are not only important for bettering communication but also for patients' mental and emotional health. A lot of the time, all patients may need is someone to be there for them and listen to them. A huge part of patient advocacy is patients having someone to explain their medical information to them as well as explain the effects and treatment options to them. Sometimes patients understand what the physician is telling them, but they do not know what that entails or are not completely told in detail what a condition or medication is. Additionally, if a patient is unsure of what to do pertaining to their medical treatment, a patient advocate may explain their options, importantly noting, that they are only explaining the facts, NOT sharing their opinion.

While every patient should have an advocate, only 70% of people do. A health advocate could be a relative, nurse, caregiver, or spouse. It is more prominent in older adults to have a health advocate and/or they are more likely to benefit from having one for medical visits and medication prescribed. This is because they are shown to have more complex and frequent medical needs.

The role of advocacy is extremely important in healthcare because it is key to building strong health systems. Patient advocacy should be implemented in all healthcare institutions because it reduces the communication gap between patients and their healthcare.

Advocating for Population Health

Population health, according to the Centers for Disease Control and Prevention (CDC), is "an interdisciplinary, customizable approach that allows health departments to connect practice to policy for change to happen locally." The study of population health focuses on the health outcomes of individuals within a certain group. Different populations often include individuals living within cities, states, or countries. However, population groups can also include people in a certain ethnic group, in the same age bracket, individuals of the same gender, professionals in an occupation, or people with a certain disability or disorder.

Population health experts seek to understand how social environments, genetics, medical care, geographic locations, behavior, and other factors have an impact on the distribution of health in a population. After specific health concerns are revealed in a studied population, communities can address those problems and improve health outcomes.

Population health has evolved as a field over the last several years and continues to grow in significance. One of the most important aspects of population health that will impact the future is understanding populations in specific health care systems. It is important for health care organizations to gain insights about their own patient populations to gather data and better serve them.

's College, Weston, Massachusetts

The Importance of the Social Determinants of Health in Diagnosing Patients

by Dima Bischoff-Hashem

According to the CDC, the social determinants of health are the "conditions in the places where people live, learn, work, and play that affect a wide range of health and quality-of-life risks and outcomes." They fall into the following categories: healthcare access and quality, education, social and community contexts, built environments, and economic stability. Healthcare access and quality are somewhat self-explanatory; access can be impacted by time, location, and financial restraints, and quality describes the effectiveness of care. Education, both formal and informal, can impact people's health through knowledge of healthy lifestyle choices. Social and community context refers to the influence those health decisions of an individual's friends, family, and community members have on their own health choices. Built environments describe a person or community's water and air quality, neighborhood safety, availability of healthy food, and access to housing and transportation. And economic stability culminates in all the proceeding categories as it affects access to healthcare, living location, and everything in between. Because social determinants of health can make individuals more prone to certain illnesses, they should be considered when diagnosing patients.

The Issues in Diagnosing Patients

A medical diagnosis is often the first step in addressing a medical condition. In order to effectively treat an illness, it is crucial to characterize it and understand its causes. The general procedure for diagnosing is as follows: an individual experiences a health concern and goes to a doctor to seek information and treatment. The doctor asks the individual about their symptoms, looks at their medical history, conducts exams, perhaps orders lab work, and then comes to a diagnosis.

Every patient has a unique set of genetic and social health factors, and as much as there are efforts to standardize the diagnosing process, doctors' perspectives and biases factor into it. The types of questions doctors ask, the direction they pursue, and the tests they order are all at their own discretion, so their lived experiences and schooling can greatly influence the final diagnosis.

Low-income populations are more commonly at risk for misdiagnosis as doctors sometimes neglect to consider the social determinants of health when diagnosing patients. For example, low-income and previously redlined neighborhoods are more likely to be polluted, a significant contributor to asthma, lung cancer, and other respiratory issues. While doctors may correctly diagnose these conditions, they may not attribute factors in a patient's environment to their onset or worsening. Therefore, doctors must investigate secondary diagnoses–additional conditions that a patient may have beyond the primary diagnosis. The secondary diagnoses may be contributing factors to the primary health concern.

A Doctor's Anecdote
Physician Renee N. Salas recounts an experience examining a girl who had been diagnosed with asthma. The patient's mother took her to Dr. Salas after diagnoses and treatment recommendations from other doctors failed to improve her condition, and her asthma worsened. Salas notes that despite being ineffective, these doctors' diagnoses and treatments followed the standard of care. In looking up her patient's home address, Salas found that she lived in a highly polluted,

previously redlined area. Familiar with the connection between asthma and air pollution, Salas immediately recognized that her patient's condition was likely connected to her living environment. Citing this experience, Salas stresses the importance of using secondary diagnoses, in this case, suspected exposure to air pollution, to contextualize and shed light on the root causes of the primary diagnosis.

Solutions for Making More Comprehensive Diagnoses

Besides pollution, medical professionals need to assess all social determinants of health. Dr. Salas' experience provides doctors with a few broad pointers to achieve this– investigating living situations and accounting for patients' environments. These are certainly important starting points, but more systemic solutions are required to address misdiagnoses large-scale. First, training on health disparities must be integrated more strongly into medical school curriculums. Currently, the standard curriculum involves courses on body and brain function, behavior, and laboratory procedures, as well as clinical practice, but no substantial course work examining the impact of the natural and built environment on health. Second, as continuing education courses are designed to educate professionals on new research and emerging treatment methods, they must be updated to emphasize the impacts of social determinants of health, as well as methods for addressing them. Other remedies include providing on-the-job training and educational materials for medical professionals that make them familiar with the health issues of the communities they serve.

Additionally, adequately addressing patients' health issues means spending enough time with them to listen to their concerns and questions and to look into their past diagnoses and living environments. Therefore, as opposed to just financial incentives for seeing a certain number of patients, healthcare systems should be modified to include incentives for patients to get well.

In addition to training for healthcare professionals, community education is critical. No matter how comprehensive, caring, and committed doctors are, they no longer make house calls. Patients know the details and changes in their lives intimately. They must also take charge of their own health. With community education, patients can make more educated connections between their health and illnesses and their environments. Armed with that information, they can better advocate for themselves in medical systems. Persistent, pervasive problems in diagnosing need multi-level solutions, from individual doctors to hospitals, health insurers, and larger societal responses.

Equal Access to Health

Many people ask how in the United States, there are still so many patients who do not have good access to our healthcare system. Why is it that in rural areas, it may take hours to get to the nearest hospital or to a doctor's office? The public health system here in the United States has been faced with this crisis for far too long, and the issue of access to quality care goes beyond our shores and is a problem throughout the world. Why do so many people believe that healthcare is a privilege for the "haves" and so difficult to get for the "have nots"? Healthcare is not a privilege. It is a right. It is the public health system that has the responsibility of ensuring that right for all Americans. That is why there are hundreds of programs being created each year to place healthcare providers in those areas where they are most needed, as well as programs to build government supported urgent care centers and small local hospitals with emergency services and maternity services where the remote rural populations need them. The public health system is fostering an alliance between the government and the major hospital systems, insisting that the hospital systems from the large cities place satellite services in the rural areas. That is why the public health system is providing incentives to new doctors, physician assistants, nurse practitioners, and rehab therapists to work in areas of the country that are less served medically.

The next section discusses some of the initiatives of bring equality of care to all parts of our country.

- Bob Kieserman

Gender Bias in Healthcare
by Liya Moges

What is Gender Bias?

According to Healthline, a major online health education portal, the direct definition of gender bias refers to "…any practice or set of beliefs that favors people of one gender over those of other genders." Gender bias tends to be a form of unconscious bias, also known as implicit bias, where the individual is usually unaware that they are attributing a certain attitude or stereotype to a certain gender. This makes gender bias a dangerous phenomenon since it can be quite difficult to observe within oneself. In the case of healthcare, gender bias specifically refers to the way an individual (usually a healthcare provider or professional) may unconsciously favor or treat a specific gender with a higher quality of care in comparison to other genders.

While such a thing as bias has no place in the healthcare profession, there have been systematic reviews and studies done on the impact of unconscious bias in the methods of healthcare delivery that provided consistent findings that such implicit bias existed. Although the severity of the bias varied among the different studies performed, there was a consensus that gender bias did indeed exist against different gendered patients by healthcare professionals.

Which Gender Receives the Most Bias?

Though no direct results are stating either women or men receive direct Gender bias as patients, there are consistent findings that women receive inadequate treatment in comparison to men, which leads to poorer outcomes. Janine

Clayton, MD, and director of the Office of Research on Women's Health at the NIH states that the possible cause of the difference in treatment dates to the disproved beliefs and outdated conventions perceived about women in earlier medical interventions. This isn't to say that men do not receive any bias as patients, however, it does prove to show that there are differences in the outcomes of medical diagnoses and treatment options provided to the different genders.

What do Gender Bias studies claim?

Many gender bias studies in medicine claim that women are less likely to receive appropriate treatments on time or in a quick manner due to assumptions by some healthcare providers that women are exaggerating their symptoms. In a study done by Josefina Robertson in Sweden in 2014, it was found that women in the emergency department, who reported symptoms and complaints of acute pain, were less likely to be given opioid painkillers (which are considered the most effective painkillers) in comparison to men. Even in the case women were prescribed the painkiller, women were recorded to have waited longer than men did to receive them. The same study observed that once in the emergency department, women waited a significantly longer time to see a doctor and were less often classified and represented as urgent cases. It seems that with several other studies, it was shown that women receive different treatment in several key departments such as pain management and cardiac care, which ultimately led to poorer health-related results.

Other gender bias studies have also found that women tended to receive more psychological-based diagnoses in comparison to men. A review completed in 2018 aimed to review gendered bias in the treatment of pain and it was noted in the data analysis of a few compiled studies that women with chronic pain were assigned psychological causes for their pain rather than physical causes. It was also reported that women with chronic pain were mistrusted and psychoanalyzed by their healthcare providers, which oftentimes resulted in a cycle of distress and increased pain in female patients. Often, it was reported that women were less likely to receive appropriate pain management medications and were more likely prescribed sedatives and antidepressants for their pain. This supports the gender bias thought that women's pain is perceived to be psychological rather than physical.

Lastly, a variety of studies also prove that women tend to face systemic related gender bias by providers due to the fact that women are generally underrepresented in clinical trials. Underrepresentation of women participants in clinical trials can make it very difficult for providers to be able to quickly assess female patients or prescribe them medications due to a lack of background information from previous studies. This underrepresentation was proven in a study published by the National Cancer Institute that found women (minority women specifically) were less likely to be included in clinical trials for cancer treatments, which leads to differences in the generalizable treatment outcomes in female populations.

How can we resolve this inequality?
Addressing something such as gender bias in healthcare requires a multi-faceted and extensively prolonged approach. One step in the right direction to approaching this problem would be having our healthcare providers receive education and training on providing equitable care to all patients and understand how to take things such as demographics and background into account when providing proper treatments. Another step would be to have healthcare systems make an effort to remove barriers to proper care such as discriminatory policies and restrictive access to gender-affirming care.

Additionally, there needs to be a greater effort from healthcare systems to provide a greater representation of women, and other minority groups and genders, in clinical trials, research studies, and policies, so that there is a larger variety of perspectives that can be put into the thought-process behind diagnoses and treatment options. By putting the effort to address the issues mentioned above, our society can work towards creating a healthcare system that works to serve and provide equitable care to all patients, regardless of their identity.

What are the Greatest Challenges in Healthcare Equity Issues?

by Hugo Amador

The years following 2019 were faced with monumental challenges in structural and systemic inequities rooted in racism and discrimination. The COVID-19 pandemic found communities without access to treatment and vaccinations. The Black Lives Matter Movement, along with the rise in Asian hate crimes, surfaced the historic disparate safety and health of Black and Asian Americans. Within two years the American public has subtly discussed the decades-long issue regarding health and healthcare disparities. A vital discussion of addressing healthcare inequities is key in narrowing the disproportionate impacts of global pandemics, in addition to the overall impacts of chronic diseases endemic to distinct populations. Albeit a proper discussion on the greatest challenges behind healthcare equity requires acknowledging which populations are affected and what feeds the issue. It may be possible that many are unaware they are a victim of this issue, therefore, in a period in time where the health of the American people can seep into the day-to-day life and well-being of individuals, tackling these challenges is pivotal in constructing a just and proper system aimed to serve its people. The overall goal of health equity does not apply only to some communities. It applies to all communities that encounter barriers on the journey to improve their health – be it a barrier against age, sex, sexual orientation, race, socioeconomic status, etc. The issue is no longer who and what is affected by these barriers, but rather how we can overcome them.

A young man in his mid-20s reported in a case study by the *New York Times* was diagnosed with Kaposi's sarcoma (KS), cancer that forms in the lining of the blood and lymph vessels – often affecting individuals with immune deficiencies such as HIV or AIDS. While undocumented, this individual along with many in the U.S. that are uninsured, face an obstacle to access and fear of the care they need. Frightened by tides of anti-immigrant sentiment, the health of undocumented patients in the U.S. is often disregarded as they are further daunted by the expense of treatment.

Thus, as shown, access to care includes more than out-of-pocket expenses. Despite an effort to mitigate disparities in the U.S., there appears to be a continuous gap in equitable access to care exacerbated by sociological and psychological factors. Health insurance status is an important factor to consider but more so are the underlying barriers that limit access to health insurance. For instance, insurance coverage, income, and available medical care resources vastly differ by ethnicity. Among Hispanic populations in the U.S., lack of public health insurance is a significant access barrier but less so for African Americans.

It is often implied that health equity is a natural successor of universal access to healthcare and health insurance. However, a study conducted by the health section of UNICEF found that models from across the globe demonstrate the success and feasibility of equity in the health sector is largely dependent on how universal access/health insurance policies are designed, defined, and implemented.

To assist in the effort of addressing racial/ethnic disparities in healthcare, many federal agencies have advised and, at times, required providers to collect racial/ethnic information on individuals. Yet, many continue to fail at reporting these demographics completely or accurately, which is vital to understanding how certain groups deviate in overall health trends and accessibility. For instance, missing race/ethnicity data in Veterans ranged from 0% to 48% in certain communities. Meanwhile, 75% of respondents who identify as Hispanic/Latino classify their race as other when asked, a collaborative study at the National Human Genome Research Institute found.

The lack of data to track which populations are, or rather are not, seeking care has aided in placing a toll against methods to make healthcare more equitable to individuals. The statistics that have been collected, however, have demonstrated that people of color, low-income individuals, and those who identify as LGBTQ+ continue to be affected by financial and mental health barriers exacerbated by the present pandemic.

The diminishing number of individuals within these demographics that seek care speaks to one issue: the lack of workforce diversity within the medical profession. One effort in addressing the diverse healthcare needs within the U.S. is training and tasking healthcare professionals within those same demographics. Many medical schools, hospitals, and clinics alike faced the difficulty of treating patients they did not relate to or sympathize with completely, thus adding an additional barrier.

With the recent Biden Administration, the president issued a series of executive orders and actions focused on advancing health equity. In March of 2021, the NIH launched the UNITE Initiative to address structural racial inequality along with the CDC's declaration of racism as a serious threat to the public's health.

Addressing these issues with policies is important to improve the underlying social and economic inequities that heighten healthcare inequities, but a broader range of initiatives from within and beyond the healthcare system is crucial in advancing equity. Increasing the availability of data, establishing incentives, accountability for equity, and recognizing discrimination are all instrumental. In addition, communicating to the demographics that are victims is influential; they must understand a key idea: before I am my sex, my gender, my class status, my race, my sexual identity, or my citizenship status, I am human. And I deserve the right to my well-being.

Rural Population and Their Health

by Alix Greenblatt

One of the more vulnerable populations, especially in countries like the United States, are those from rural areas. This is not specific to farmers, but they are not excluded from the conversation either. The biggest reason the rural population is one of the more susceptible populations to health risks is due to their isolation from many health service areas–hospitals, physician offices, healthcare clinics, pharmacies, etc. Some communities are luckier than others as they may have a medical facility nearby. In this case, nearby would mean 10-15 minutes of driving. However, for some communities, calling an ambulance may take over 30 minutes, if they're lucky.

Along with geographic isolation, other health disparities amongst the rural community include (but are not excluded to) lower socioeconomic status, higher rates of health risk behaviors, limited access to healthcare specialists, and limited job opportunities. Another risk factor is rural residents are less likely to have health insurance coverage provided by employers. Additionally, they may not be covered by Medicaid either. With 15% of the United States population living in rural areas, around five million people are affected by these health disparities.

In 2021, 39.21% of the world's population resided in rural areas. Papua New Guinea has the highest percentage of rural residents in the world with Bermuda having the lowest. The struggle for healthcare that plagues the rural residents in the United States also occurs in other parts of the world. The health disparities mentioned above are equally applied to other parts of the world, some having the additional risk of climate change and water accessibility. These risk factors go hand in hand. Climate change has been known for causing droughts around the world, causing the accessibility of clean/safe water to decline.

Are there solutions to this issue? Possibly, but they won't be easy or necessarily feasible. The first option for this would be building more healthcare facilities in areas where rural populations reside. A newly popular/important concept for healthcare–telemedicine could pave a smooth and strong path for rural communities to receive the health advice and services they need. Increasing the incentive for healthcare providers to move toward rural communities would not just benefit the community but those who would be working for them as well. In order to implement those incentives, federal governments will need to be more involved. Healthcare is a human right, according to the Universal Declaration of Human Rights (the right est. in 1966).

Collaboration is key and if this can be achieved with federal governments, the future for rural communities and their healthcare rights will improve.

Why is Diversity in Medicine So Important?

by Michelle Powell

Diversity in the healthcare system has a complicated history. From surgical experimentations performed on African American women without anesthesia to medical devices, specifically, being created for African Americans, the medical field has become, unknowingly, racist. This not only impacts African Americans but minority races and religions that feel targeted based on their identity.

Why is it a problem?
During my undergraduate years, I remember reading a text for a class that described how African Americans were believed to have a decreased pain tolerance than Caucasian people. Realistically, it is not true, but I was horrified to read that this false belief has been held strongly in the past and even been mentioned in medical school textbooks. While it is not the fault of the private and public institutions that educate young people, racism is deep-rooted in America's social, political, and economic structures, as Harvard Health mentions. Because of this, it is hard to steer clear of a problem that has become a part of society itself and to realize its impacts.

As America has become diverse and understood its past mistakes, they have comprehended why it is not okay to treat patients unequally. Doctors, at the beginning of their careers, take an oath to treat their patients equally. While this is acceptable to live and work by, it still does not take care of the implicit bias or racism that occurs every day in doctor's offices or hospitals. Minorities are known for receiving a decreased amount of "technological and surgical procedures and routine healthcare preventive service", as was reported by Stanford Medical. Minorities will then not be able to gain the appropriate help they deserve and instead be pushed aside because their doctors do not believe their problem is substantial or serious enough. This causes many people to become vulnerable and their undiagnosed health situations to worsen.

Developing Distrust
On the other hand, patients who are denied appropriate healthcare may develop distrust in their doctors and the medical system. They, moreover, may look toward unconventional healthcare methods that may worsen their conditions and, in the end, put their lives at risk. As a future physician, I do not desire any of my future patients to receive unfamiliar health procedures from an unlicensed physician or to put them in harm's way.

So How Do We Solve the Problem of Racism?
I believe racism should be the first and foremost concern of physicians, nurses, and other providers because they can control their biases and actions toward their patients. Most importantly, medical personnel need to start practicing and modeling tolerance, respect, open-mindedness, and peace. Change starts with those that desire and have a will for it, and I believe the medical field is no exception. Another way to prevent racism is to encourage young people and minorities who have a desire to enter the medical profession to pursue it. By helping minorities and educating future generations on diversity and racism, they can help others who make mistakes and make their patients feel more confident going into their doctor's office. Minority physicians are more likely to care for minorities, the poor, and uninsured persons additionally in underserved communities. Through this, they can increase healthcare for them, too.

As a minority and future physician, I dream that every minority will be able to feel confident and comfortable in any healthcare setting, whatever their racial, ethnic, religious, etc. background. I am blessed to not have experienced racism in a healthcare setting and want my future patients to have similar experiences.

Examining the Causes Behind Black Health Disparities

by Elika Oakley

Social determinants of health are important to help understand the underlying causes of the health disparities that African Americans experience. Social, economic, and political resources and structures, also known as social determinants, are responsible for a larger portion of health disparities because they impact one's ability to buffer disease. It is also important to understand that there is not one social determinant that can describe health disparities for African Americans. Health disparities are caused by a collection of social determinants that interact with each other. In this article, we will examine how education, employment, and poverty play a role in health disparities for Black patients.

Fundamental Causes: Education, Employment, Poverty

Although the death gap between whites and Black Americans has narrowed since 1999, health disparities continue to be the leading catalyst of death for Black individuals over their lifespan. Particularly, Black Americans had higher rates in the leading causes of death (Cunningham et al., 2017). This can be linked to "fundamental causes", such as low educational attainment, unemployment, and poverty. In a study done by Cunningham et al. (2017), researchers found that when compared to their white counterparts, Black Americans of all age groups were more likely to have less than 12 years of education, to be unemployed, and live below the poverty line. These factors have compounding effects on each other making it even harder for Black Americans to achieve good health in these circumstances.

Education

Education is a vital tool because it allows individuals to advance their knowledge and gain new opportunities. There are many connections to how education affects health. In a study analyzed by Braveman and Gottlieb (2014), researchers showed that women with lower educational attainment rates live shorter, and the lower a pregnant mother's education level is the lower chance an infant has of surviving. When people are more educated, they have greater access to resources to help navigate the health care system and health complications.

Employment

Employment also plays a huge role in health because it generates income and provides benefits, such as health insurance. Income is necessary to help pay for health care, prescriptions, and medical bills. Employment benefits, such as health insurance, are necessary to help lower the out-of-pocket price so that people can afford the care they need. Unfortunately, Black Americans are more likely to be unemployed compared to their white counterparts, which hinders their access to the resources that are necessary to afford medical care––income and health insurance. Even when Black Americans are employed, many of them still struggle to get access to adequate salaries and health insurance. There is a "disproportionate percentage of African Americans who
work in jobs that do not provide health insurance" (Copeland, 2005). This impacts their ability to access and afford medical care.

Poverty

Living at or below the poverty line has damaging effects on Black Americans; health at all stages of life. In a study by Fiscella & Williams (2004), the researchers show that children living in poverty have higher sudden infant death,

child abuse, asthma, developmental delays, and overall poor health. The study continues to show that adolescents who live in poverty experience higher
rates of pregnancies, sexually transmitted diseases, depression, obesity, and suicide. By adulthood, Black Americans in poverty experience premature chronic morbidity and have higher rates of death across the spectrum of causes (Fiscella & Williams, 2004).

Conclusion

These fundamental causes lead to poor health outcomes for Black Americans because they limited their human capital and ability to get access to health-promoting resources. In combination, the lack of education, employment, and living in poverty can lead to higher stress levels and allostatic load. This contributes to high rates of hypertension, cardiovascular disease, and cumulative physiological effects--on top of the negative health outcomes that already come with each fundamental cause individually.

Educational attainment, employment, and poverty are not the only social barriers that are causing health disparities for Black patients. There are several other factors that play a role, and determining the exact social determinants of health is complex. Although the causal pathways of every Black Americans' health disparity may not be known, it is still important to try to reduce these disparities because health is a basic human right.

AAPI Health Disparities and Recommended Action

by Ashley Mui

AAPI, or Asian American Pacific Islander, communities are one of the fastest-growing populations in the United States. In 2020, the U.S. Census recorded that the AAPI population constituted 6% or 20 million of the United States population. The umbrella term, AAPI, refers to the many subgroups of individuals with roots from over 30 countries. Yet despite their rapidly growing populations, Asian Americans and Pacific Islanders have yet to observe representation in health data and research.

From what we do know, however, AAPI populations disproportionately suffer from a number of diseases. Among Asian Americans, cancer and cardiovascular disease are the leading causes of death. Asian Americans report the highest incidence and mortality rates of liver and stomach cancers despite their preventability, which is linked to Hepatitis B prevalence in Asian American populations. Cases of Hepatitis B in Asian American communities are staggering; they account for over half of all chronic Hepatitis B diagnoses.

Diabetes is also prevalent, with an estimated 20% and 32% of Asian Americans suffering from diabetes and pre-diabetes, respectively. AAPI health statistics continually beg the question: *Why do so many health disparities exist in AAPI populations?*

One of the main root causes of AAPI health disparities lies in health insurance. In 2021, 6% of Asian people and 11% of NHOPI (Native Hawaiian and Other Pacific Islander) people were uninsured. Although the proportion of uninsured Asian individuals was lower than that of their white counterparts with uninsured rates of 7%, NHOPI communities are still disproportionately affected. Statistically, AAPI subgroups show socioeconomic differences – another leading contributor to health insurance coverage disparities. For example, Asian subgroups have a higher degree of educational attainment than NHOPI subgroups. Even within these subgroups, there are differences. While 87% of Taiwanese individuals receive a bachelor's degree or higher, only 18% of Laotion people achieve the same. In NHOPI communities, 28% of Chamorro people receive college degrees compared to 6% of Marshallese people. Lower educational attainment levels are one of the causes associated with lower socioeconomic status as well as health insurance coverage. On the other hand, AAPI communities may also experience differences in socioeconomic status promoted by citizenship and/or visa status. Individuals with work visas in comparison to those entering the country with asylee or refugee status are more likely to attain higher median household incomes. Conversely, entering the United States without a work visa may also contribute to lower median household incomes. Access to health insurance is key to positive outcomes. Uninsured patients in the United States are less likely to receive preventative services for chronic conditions often caused by genetic predispositions. What is more – children are the largest population at risk, as they are unable to receive critical health services during developmental periods. This only perpetuates cycles of minority health disparities in the long run. Studies also show that access to health insurance simultaneously increases access and usage of health services.

Asian American groups are also commonly confronted with the longstanding issue of language barriers. In the United States, almost 25% of AAPI students are considered "Limited English Proficient" or live in households where their parents have limited English proficiency. In total, around 34% of

Asian Americans are deemed to have limited English proficiency. The term "limited English proficiency," commonly referred to as LEP, describes anyone over the age of 5 who speaks English "less than very well." In the United States, the majority of LEP speakers are Hispanic or Asian. However, due to linguistic diversity among Asian speakers, it is more difficult to accommodate Asian LEP individuals in comparison to Hispanic LEP individuals, whose dominant language is Spanish (spoken by around 99% of the Hispanic LEP population). The impacts of such language barriers are two-fold. First, population studies done on Asian populations are hindered by failing to represent the minority subgroups that are unable to participate in such studies due to a lack of language representation. Without proper accommodation of LEP speakers in such subgroups, entire populations are skewed out of significant health data rendering. Currently, health data on LEP and non-English speaking Asians severely underestimate the totality of Asian health vulnerabilities. Language barriers also carry the detriment of health service inaccessibility. In a study by Yuri Jang and Miyong T. Kim, being an Asian LEP individual increased the probability of not having a usual place for healthcare by 2.09 times, inability to receive a regular check-up by 1.69 times, having unmet medical needs by 1.89 times, and having communication issues in healthcare settings by 4.95 times. These healthcare-related challenges encapsulate only a few of the many determinants that deter Asian American populations from accessing adequate healthcare and even quality of life.

Unfortunately, our previous discussion only covers surface-level issues that plague AAPI health outcomes. What lies beneath the surface of health disparities today are stereotypes. Although stereotypes targeting AAPI populations may not specifically pertain to healthcare, they are strong proponents of negative beliefs that eventually cause a trickle-down effect on health outcomes. Anti-Asian sentiment dates back decades

– common examples include Sinophobia, the "yellow peril," and the "fu manchu" stereotypes of the mid-19th and 20th centuries. Paradoxically, Asian communities are also under threat by the model minority myth, which portrays Asian individuals as "high-performing" and assimilated into American society, effectively ignoring their struggles as a whole in comparison to other minorities. These two sociological phenomena in combination lead to the erasure, otherization, and scapegoating of Asians, as this country observed during the COVID-19 pandemic. Moreover, it ignores the statistics that prove various subgroups in the AAPI population experience poverty at higher-than-average levels. The conceptualization of AAPI individuals in the United States has alarming implications for health data. Mainly, it groups AAPI people into the same category without observing or studying the diversity of populations about their genetic ancestry, immigration histories, or socioeconomic statuses. Without disaggregated data on AAPI subgroups, the healthcare system is unable to develop a nuanced understanding of AAPI health disparities and barriers to care. Painting AAPI people as "model minorities" also has unintended consequences for mental health outcomes. Particularly among younger Asian people, academic success is highly prioritized and can lead to intense stress, anxiety, and/or depression. AAPI people are also culturally conditioned to minimize conversations surrounding mental health due to the stigmatization of mental health issues being viewed as a risk to one's standing as a "model minority." A study performed by Kelly Guanhua Yang et al. indicates that Asian Americans access mental health treatment at less than half the rate of other racial groups despite rising cases of serious mental illness, major depressive episodes, and suicidal thoughts, plans, or attempts.

Recommended Action

There is no one surefire way to fully address all AAPI health disparities, but there are certain steps this country can take to ensure gradually better health outcomes for all AAPI populations.

To first tackle the issue of unrepresentative data, national health organizations must prioritize the inclusion of non-English speaking and LEP individuals in AAPI populations. To do so, translators or assistants who speak less common languages should be utilized during population studies to accommodate those currently unable to participate. Workforce diversity is thus also highly important for the medical and health research fields, as it will encourage not only the breaking down of language barriers in population studies but also the be the betterment of cultural humility in healthcare. Successful exchanges between medical providers and AAPI patients include the use of language interpreters, readable patient materials, and facilitators for navigating patient services.

Governmental action must also be taken to increase accessibility to healthcare through the expansion of affordable insurance. Such a proposition has been pitched to the United States government repeatedly, but li le action has been taken. Until affordable healthcare can be secured, the medical community must begin the process of educating AAPI communities, especially those immigrating to the United States, on their current options. According to AJSoCal CEO Connie Chung Joe, many AAPI families who are LEP, uninsured, or undocumented are uneducated on the benefits of programs such as Covered California or MediCal, in California. On top of community education, cultural humility and cultural competency must be normalized and standardized in healthcare. Understanding patients' culture as a part of their process of care is integral to improving experiences with medical professionals, the likelihood of seeking medical treatment, and the overall inclusion of AAPI individuals in medicine.

Increased emphasis on AAPI enrollment in population studies is likely to improve the current state of AAPI representation in medicine. Previously overlooked and underemphasized health issues will come to light – and AAPI communities will need resources to combat generational health determinants. Language inclusivity and enhancement of health insurance policies are only a few of the ways AAPI health disparities can be addressed, but they are a start.

The Foreignness of Disease

by Hugo Amador

The 20th and 21st centuries met the United States with revolutionary, innovative socio-political transformations tangent with new advancements in medical diagnosis and treatment. However, the rise in anti-immigrant propaganda in the mid-1950s propagated a narrative, or question rather, against immigrant populations and their health here in America: are immigrants backtracking our success by bringing disease to the United States?

Despite the transcendence toward more effective measures to treat acute and chronic disease, immigrants in the United States have continually been associated with contagion. Anti-immigrant rhetoric regarding endemic diseases among these groups has developed etiological stigmas of physical and societal ills.

The dawn of the 1980s faced the rise of the AIDS epidemic in the United States. In that same decade, amidst public demands and pressures, the Senate and President Ronald Regan passed the 1986 Immigration Reform and Control Act. This legislation made it illegal for employers to hire illegal immigrants and further fueled distrust against all immigrant groups alike, illegal, or not. The growing fears of the AIDS epidemic intertwined with distrust against immigrant groups led the public eye to direct blame and risk toward immigrant individuals.

At the time, those seeking refugee status in the United States had to submit to an HIV test, while those wishing to take up permanent residence that tested positive for HIV were banned. Dr. Paul Spiegel, director of the Center for

Humanitarian Health at Johns Hopkins School of Public Health, said, "There is no evidence to show that migrants are spreading [any kind] of disease. That is a false argument used to keep migrants out."

Dr. Spiegel was one among a group of commissioners who tackled a two-year analysis of migration trends and models to determine whether immigration into the United States was spreading disease. In their study, they found that immigrants are far less likely than other groups to suffer or die from the more prominent causes of death in the United States–heart disease, cancer, and respiratory diseases. Even among diseases like HIV, data from Dr. Spiegel's project formulated that they generally remain enclosed within immigrant communities and stray away from the overall population.

An additional monumental study published in The Lancet concluded a worldwide immigration study that dates as far back as 1994, which supported that immigration does not bring new diseases into host countries or spread old diseases. Most of those migrating to the United States originate from countries that have higher vaccination rates compared to the U.S. for all forms of diseases, including measles, diphtheria, and polio. In fact, both studies have concluded that immigrant populations correlate with healthier host countries.

The Obesity Pandemic
by Angela DeMondo

Chronic illnesses have been on the rise since the age of civilized society began, slowly becoming a conceptualized modern-day pandemic costing the healthcare system billions. Though it is a chronic illness in and of itself, obesity raises the possibility of developing additional lifelong illnesses. There is a distinction to be made between being overweight and being obese. More than 35% of people in the US are considered obese and are a high health risk, according to a study from Harvard University. Fighting obesity takes time, effort, discipline, and a plan to do it.

What is obesity?
The general American population associates the term "obesity" with a negative body image. There is, however, a greater understanding of obesity that goes beyond what most people know. The World Health Organization (WHO) defines a person as being obese if their body mass index is greater than 30% and overweight if it is between 25% and 29%. Obesity limits a person's ability to live a normal life by diminishing endurance, limiting movement of the spine and major joints, reducing muscle strength, limiting the capacity to keep prolonged fixed postures, limiting breathing capacity, and limiting visual control. Several factors contribute to the development of obesity, including genetics, environmental factors, underlying health conditions, and medication usage. The major cause of obesity, however, is attributed to excessive

calorie consumption and a sedentary lifestyle, which result in $147 billion in annual healthcare expenses. According to a study by the Centers for Disease Control and Prevention (CDC), obesity is more likely to develop in people over the age of 40. Additionally, the study found that the age group between 20 and 39 years old accounts for approximately 40% of obesity cases. Low-income families have been found to have significantly higher rates of obesity, primarily attributed to the limited access to healthy dietary options and the prevalence of affordable junk food. Obesity not only diminishes the quality of life for those it affects, but it also presents significant health risks.

The Obesity Risks for Chronic Disease Development

According to CDC and American Family Care, 2022, the following are some of the risks for developing chronic disease as a result of obsesity:

- **Heart Disease**: the leading chronic illness in the United States with a high $363 billion annual healthcare cost

- **Heart Attack or Stroke**: ranks fourth in chronic illness reports, costing $36 billion in healthcare

- **Type 2 Diabetes:** ranks as the sixth most common chronic illness, incurring $327 billion in healthcare costs

Other Health Risks as stated by the CDC 2022
- **Osteoarthritis**
- **Sleep apnea and breathing problems**
- **Cancer**
- **Sudden Death**
- **High blood pressure**
- **High or Low Cholesterol**

Treatment Options

Though obesity has detrimental impacts on health, there are several treatment options to choose from. Considering that poor diet and inactivity are the leading causes of obesity, dietary changes, and exercise are the foundation to becoming healthy. Medication weight loss alternatives that the Mayo Clinic has listed are Bupropion-Naltrexone, Liraglutide, Orlistat, and Semaglutide. Procedures that lower the amount of food a person's stomach can hold, like endoscopic sleeve gastroplasty and intragastric balloon, can help with weight loss. There are also surgical options, such as gastric bypass, which cuts a section of the intestine so that food and drinks go straight from the pouch into this section of the intestine; gastric sleeve, which cuts a section of the stomach; and adjustable gastric banding, which creates pouches in the stomach to limit food intake. Despite the negative impact of obesity on an individual's overall well-being, there are various options to effectively address and improve this condition, preventing further long-term effects.

In Conclusion

The prevalence of chronic illnesses, notably obesity, is linked to the development of various long-term health conditions across the country. Long-term health issues such as diabetes and heart disease significantly reduce an individual's quality of life while also increasing the individual's chance of unfavorable health impacts. There are numerous treatment options available to help reduce the harmful impacts of obesity. Obesity is a health issue that can be reversed.

PART THREE: LOOKING AT THE FUTURE

Throughout this book, we have addressed some of the current issues in public health and suggested some new needs based on an ever-changing population. In this final section, we address in greater detail some of the issues that need to be considered in post-pandemic America. The first issue is the threat of corporate healthcare taking over the healthcare delivery system and how the public health system needs to address this issue. The second commentary is a much more positive one. It looks at some of the successes that have come about from the diligence and advocacy of public health practitioners to strengthen global health initiatives. Finally, the last essay looks at what is needed by Americans from their public health system.

- Bob Kieserman

The Commercialization of Our Medical Institutions

by Olivia Arkell

The advancements made in the last couple of decades have made medicine and its related practices and relationships incredibly complex. The healthcare industry has become commercialized over the last few decades, something we've feared happening. This has led to ethical concerns related to medical practices and financial arrangements. These concerns were anticipated by the American Medical Association in 1957.

For-profit corporatization of healthcare poses many ethical concerns. This has led to unethical relationships and arrangements involving the physicians who are prescribing drugs, those who are conducting the research, and companies who are providing the drugs. This is problematic because it can promote incentives, enticements, and compensation for particular patterns of practice.

The American Medical Association (AMA) worked toward avoiding these turning medical practices into business affairs. The AMA tried to nurture this trust by developing codes and guidelines in 1957 that would prevent the medical profession from becoming a business. To make these expectations more concrete, the AMA declared that medical judgment should be free of financial interest: "A physician should not dispose of his services under terms or conditions that tend to interfere with or impair the free and complete exercise of his medical judgment and skill or tend to cause a deterioration of the quality of medical care" (Shwartz & Sharpe, 2010). The AMA expected physicians to refrain from advertising and financial arrangements with drug and device manufacturers; they heavily pushed for the separation of prescribing pharmaceutical drugs from the sale of the drug itself.

However, in the era of commercialization and pursuit of profit, our medical institutions have inevitably built such relationships with related affiliations. Although arranging a profitable relationship between a physician and a pharmaceutical institute violates many of the AMA Code of Ethics, it still occurs. Disobeying these standards by valuing pharmaceutical enticements and financial compensation over the treatment of the patient is an indisputable unethical act. Furthermore, it completely disregards the pivotal virtues a physician ought to possess. These arrangements tend to undermine devotion to the profession, making it more difficult for physicians to balance the main objective of the profession and the financial compensation that comes with it. As shown, a physician's financial relationship with pharmaceutical firms is a massive ethical concern that has raised important questions about the virtues of a good physician. Physicians are expected to treat their clients with advanced medical knowledge, virtue, and practical wisdom. Interference of personal financial gain will inevitably skew the way these physicians treat their clients due to underlying motivations.

The medical industry's involvement in financial, organizational, and legal arrangements in drug research, marketing, and regulation is worthy of consideration. These arrangements tend to weaken institutions' proficiency in advancing medical knowledge, drug safety, and public health. This decreases the integrity of pharmaceutical institutions and the physicians involved. In the article, "The Effects of Pharmaceutical Firm Enticements on Physician Prescribing Patterns (1992)," it was made apparent that some physicians lack the willingness to further advance their knowledge on certain topics and drugs. When incentives are offered, this leads to a tendency to ignore important factors that physicians wouldn't typically ignore. Even more surprisingly, some physicians were inclined to prescribe these incentivized drugs even after given a limited analysis of data. The lack of objective data made these drugs look more appealing which helped them confirm their desire to prescribe them, regardless of if they were receiving enticements or incentives.

Not only can these corrupt relations negatively influence the treatment of patients, but even more concerning, the entire research and clinical trial of prospective drugs. Arrangements involving a physician and a pharmaceutical firm are one unethical dilemma, but institutional corruption involving drug research itself is a whole other dilemma. The relationships between physicians and pharmaceutical firms are also interconnected with pharmaceutical firms' relationship with research and development organizations.

The primary problem isn't necessarily physicians' virtues and ethics, rather it is an implication of the structures of our organizations. Physicians' ethical virtues (or lack thereof) are part of the problem, but they are also a product of the problem. This has contributed to the commercialization of our healthcare system and the relationships that promote it. With that being said, the systems in place are ultimately the main culprit, not the individual physicians who might lack ethical and virtuous standards.

Although it may be unethical for physicians to participate in such arrangements, in some instances the structures they are under don't make it easy to resist these temptations. It is clear the pursuit of profit is present in our current culture. We are faced with corruption and incentives on different levels and within different intuitions. Changing system organization and financial interests in the medical setting might seem like the practical way to go about this. However, one could argue this is unattainable given the pace of development we are facing and the culture we are in. Since we are in a profit-driven era, some find it much more practical to adapt to the demands and climate around commercialization. We might not be able to completely eradicate temptations within the profession, but we must discover ways in which we can alter our systems in an innovative and creative way that is compatible with the society we live in. Finding a way to make these relationships ethical is crucial if we want to sustain the integrity of our healthcare systems and the physicians that are employed by them.

A New Model of Medical Practice

by Bob Kieserman

Recently, a doctor challenged me on my approach to the provider-patient relationship. He said that I am much too hard on the doctors and that the suggestions that I make to patients in my role of Executive Director of The Power of the Patient Project on what they have a right to expect when visiting their doctor are not fair, and much too unrealistic in the world of corporate medicine. The doctor pointed out to me, that while he totally agrees with what I believe patients should expect from their doctors and their support staffs, corporate medicine simply does not allow most doctors to do the things I am suggesting, and that we should not fault the doctors, but rather, the big hospital systems for whom they work. He told me we need to give the doctors and their staff a break. I thanked him for his thoughts and realized that he is right. As patients, we have the right to expect certain things from our healthcare providers, but in many cases, their hands are tied, and they are really doing the best they can under the circumstances.

The way it once was

It's been a while, but I remember when almost every doctor in America owned his or her office with a small staff, often just a nurse and a receptionist who was typically the doctor's spouse. Many of the offices were scattered throughout the neighborhoods in both small towns and larger cities, and others were in office buildings near neighborhood hospitals where all of the suites were occupied by doctors. I am talking about a time when in many towns, there was a hospital in almost every major neighborhood. Most of the waiting rooms in the offices were small and quite quaint, and your wait to see the doctor was typically very short, but the time spent with the doctor often lasted 20 minutes or longer. I remember that when I had a doctor's appointment, I was often the only one in the waiting room because that was the way the doctor scheduled patients. If I was ever sick growing up, the doctor would even come to my house. It was aptly called a house call, and doctors had one or two days a week when they routinely made them. I really miss those days. I know a lot of doctors do also.

The major change in healthcare services

In 1990, there were 6,650 hospitals in the United States. In 2016, there were 5,530. That is because around 2010, a new chapter in healthcare management began to take place. Between 2010 and 2017, hospital systems were formed with major hospitals in various regions of the country buying smaller hospitals and/or merging with similar size hospitals to form large regional healthcare systems. And as part of the game plan of the hospital systems to become the major healthcare supplier, doctors in private practice were approached to sell their practices to the healthcare systems. At first, many doctors (especially older very established private practitioners) resisted, but the offers by the hospital systems were so lucrative that the doctors accepted the offers. Some of the older doctors retired at that point, while others who wanted to continue to practice medicine became employees for the first time in their medical careers. For those doctors, life became very different. No longer were the doctors making decisions about the business operations of their practices. That now became the responsibility of the hospital systems who took over. The doctors were employees, and their job was just to practice medicine. The hospital systems took care of everything else. At the same time, the hospital systems placed many protocols on the doctors and their staff like how much time a doctor should spend with a patient, how many patients the staff needs to schedule in a certain day, whether a patient should see a doctor or a physician assistant or a certified nurse practitioner, and other rules that became universal of all system-owned offices. At the same time, for-profit healthcare corporations who owned hospitals and created their own network of employed doctors were growing. Over the past two years, the hospital systems and these for-profit corporations have continued to grow even larger, but the big question is whether this change has benefited the patient or not.

A recent study by the Physician Advocacy Institute and Avalere Health found that the pandemic actually accelerated this trend of corporate medicine acquiring physician practices with over 25,000 physicians leaving their private practices and joining these hospitals and companies since the pandemic began. It is estimated that in the beginning of 2021, nearly 70% of physicians were employed with just 3 out of 10 doctors still practicing independently.

The doctors are not happy
Late last year, the Physicians Advocacy Institute sent an open letter to members of Congress to warn against this "major shift toward the corporatization of healthcare". According to the open letter, if Congress did not take action to monitor the activities of these big hospital systems and prevent them from reducing the clinical autonomy of doctors to provide high-quality, cost-effective care for patients, this could have major implications for the overall American healthcare system and affect the welfare of patients across the country. This is the real issue with the change to corporate medicine – that doctors have lost the ability to practice medicine as they were trained to do and to make clinical decisions for the good of the patient, not for the good of the companies that now own their offices.

How this affects patients

It has been said that the big hospital systems and the for-profit healthcare companies have pressured their employed doctors to see patients more often for followup visits, order more tests that the third party insurance companies will pay for, push for virtual visits rather than live in office visits (since they can charge the same for a virtual visit as they do for an in-office visit), and scheduling more appointments with the PA or the CNP instead of the doctor because they are seeking high financial returns in reimbursements and fees for service. Patients have also complained that doctors spend more time looking at the computer during a visit than talking to the patient and examining them. This is due to new protocols connected with the use of electronic medical records. Because many offices are scheduling three patients or more for the same appointment time, the doctor is rushed and no longer fully examining a patient. I have come to learn and appreciate that the doctors are not happy with the situation. They are doing the best they can, but they know they are not giving their patients the same personal attention they once did. In some cases, this new way of practicing medicine has caused physician burnout with many excellent doctors retiring earlier than planned or leaving medicine altogether and getting into a different career path. For many older patients, in particular, the doctors who have cared for them for decades are deciding they have had enough, are retiring, and leaving the older patients to find new doctors and start new relationships late in life.

What can patients do?

There are two major things patients can do to help the situation. The first is understand and verbally support your doctors. Tell them how much you appreciate them; tell them that you understand they are under new pressures that they never had before and try to be less demanding on what you know should be, but just can't be right now. The other thing that patients can do is to let the hospital systems and/or the healthcare companies know that you value your doctors and that they need to give as much autonomy to the doctors as possible for the benefit of their patients. Patients can make a difference. Large systems and corporations are big on surveys. They send them out all of the time, especially after an office or virtual visit. Be honest about your experiences and let them know that doctors need to be able to practice medicine with full decision-making powers, such as deciding what is best for the patient including what tests need to be ordered, what specialists they need to see, how often they need to return for followup visits, and how necessary it is for certain medications to be prescribed or not prescribed.

Together, we may be able to change the way our healthcare is being delivered. But we need to be proactive with the systems and let them know how we really feel and be understanding and supportive of our healthcare providers and let them know that we want change.

Global Health Successes

by Caitlin Laska

To begin our look at global health successes, we must understand what global health is. Global health studies the health of all populations worldwide. While the burdens of disease for the average American may look different from the average Brazilian, Pakistani, or Jordanian, global health and its accomplishments impact us all, and it is a united fight to better health worldwide. We have already come such a long way in global health. According to the UN Populations Division, the average life expectancy worldwide was 46.5 in 1955. In 2022, it was 71.7 years. While it is true that medical advancements have saved countless lives, public health advancements are also responsible. According to a 2022 study from Harvard researchers, 44% of improved life expectancy can be attributed to public health. Let's take a deeper dive into some of the greatest areas of global health achievements and examples of success stories that have saved and improved millions of lives.

Reduction in Child and Maternal Mortality

Over the past few decades, there has been substantial progress made in reducing maternal and child mortality worldwide. According to the World Health Organization, the total number of child deaths under 5 years of age has declined from 12.8 million in 1990 to 5 million in 2021. Further, the number of neonatal (children under one month) deaths has dramatically decreased from 5.2 million in 1990 to 2.3 million in 2021. Maternal mortality rates have also significantly declined by 34% since 2000. Since the majority of these deaths occur in Sub-Saharan Africa, the region has been an area of focus for improving global health. One of the main contributions to lowering the mortality rate has been increasing the number of births in hospitals and clinics to around 80% of all births worldwide. The World Health Organization states that providing newborn care and identifying risks in newborns is critical to the health and safety of the babies. In addition, providers can identify and treat any life-threatening issues during birth.

Before any intervention, Malawi had one of the worst maternal and child mortality rates in the world. According to the World Health Organization, 2.78% of women died during childbirth. In addition, the neonatal mortality rate was approximately 30 per 1,000 live births. However, former President Joyce Banda, president from 2012 to 2014, created a plan to get more women into hospitals and away from traditional birth attendants. In Malawi, traditional birth attendants had no formal medical training and were not equipped to deal with the complications that can occur with childbirth. It is important to note that former President Banda was not the first to attempt this. Back in 2007, there was a national ban on giving birth at home. However, many Malawians ignored it. Instead of going against the local culture, former President Banda created the new concept of Secret Mothers who are responsible for monitoring the mother's health, providing access to prenatal and postnatal care, and ensuring that the mother delivers her baby in a health facility. However, it is not easy to create a public health initiative without local support. Former President Banda had to work with local chiefs to gain the trust of the communities. By combining local tradition and modern medicine, thousands of lives were saved. Now, according to WHO, the maternal mortality rate is 0.38% and the neonatal mortality rate is 19.77

per 1,000 live births. While there is still a lot of work needed to lower these rates, Malawi is a clear example of the extraordinary public health achievements in maternal and child mortality.

Vaccines

Immunizations have been one of the most successful public health interventions in the past 50 years. Scientists now know how to prevent lethal diseases that used to ravage the world. We have even seen global health victories from vaccines in the eradication of polio, eradicated in the U.S. in 1979, to smallpox. Successful vaccines are developed to protect against many human pathogens such as influenza, measles, yellow fever, and more. However, their success is not only dependent on successful science but also successful public health. In order for the vaccines to be effective, public health officials must persuade people to get the vaccine and provide vaccines to everyone no matter the location. We have already seen great success with this. In 2019, according to the World Health Organization, global vaccination coverage was at 86%. However, it is important to note that COVID-19 lockdowns, vaccine hesitancy, and vaccine inequality have severely impacted the success of overall vaccinations, lowering the global coverage to 81% in 2021.

One prime example of global health success when it comes to vaccines can be seen in eradicating Smallpox in Bangladesh. Smallpox is an acute and contagious disease that presents in a painful rash all over the body. According to the World Health Organization, the deadliest strain, Variola Major, killed almost one-third of its victims. Those who survived were scarred and sometimes blinded. In 1971, Bangladesh declared that it had eradicated smallpox from its borders. However, it was later discovered that there were indeed still cases present due to civil unrest. In the spring of 1975, health workers started using a house-to-house survey method that had been previously successful in India. In that effort, 12,000 health workers checked 1,000 houses asking residents if they knew anyone with smallpox symptoms. To increase willingness to participate, people were given the equivalent of 6 dollars if they reported an undetected case of smallpox. Although the campaign seemed impossible, over 12 million homes were surveyed, and the initiative reduced the number of cases to 150 in only a few months. Four months later, the region was declared free of smallpox. We often credit public health officials and medical providers with success in these cases; however, the eradication would not have been possible without the support of local volunteers.

Malaria
While not seen until recently in the U.S., malaria is a significant public health concern for countries near the equator. Malaria can be fatal and is caused by a parasite that infects mosquitoes. When a mosquito bites a human, it transmits the parasite. People who get malaria are often sick with high fevers, shaking, chills, and flu-like symptoms. According to the World Health Organization, nearly half of the world's population is at risk for malaria. Each year, there are an estimated 247 million malaria cases worldwide, which is equivalent to over two-thirds of the U.S. population. On the other hand, there are prevention measures available to stop the spread of malaria. Since the disease is spread through mosquitoes, the best method of prevention is to eliminate

contact with mosquitoes. The CDC suggests wearing long-sleeved shirts and pants, insect repellant, and mosquito nets. According to the World Health Organization, these interventions have already prevented 1.5 billion malaria cases and 7.6 million deaths since 2000.

There have been many malaria success stories over the years, however, Ghana's malaria prevention campaign sets it apart. In 2016, the Ghanaian government started a campaign in Northern Ghana to stop the spread of malaria. Northern Ghana is significantly poorer and more rural than Southern Ghana, leaving it at a higher risk of malaria. According to the 2022 Ghana Demographic and Health Survey, malaria rates are three times higher in rural areas than in urban areas. In addition, approximately 13 in 100 people in Northern Ghana will get malaria each year. As a result, an intervention was immediately needed. The Malaria Prevention Program began in May 2016 with a country-wide campaign to distribute insecticide-treated nets to 1.2 million children at over 14,000 schools in Central and Northern Ghana over the course of 10 days. The event was led by the National Malaria Control Program of the Ghana Health Service in partnership with the U.S. President's Malaria Initiative. According to an article in the International Journal of Environmental Research and Public Health, malaria cases account for 40% of all outpatient visits to hospitals in Ghana, resulting in countless school days missed. This severely impacts Ghana's economic potential as well by setting behind student education and time available to work. By implementing this campaign, Ghana hopes to reduce malaria mortality rates and incidences of illness. While there appear to be no updates on the program specifically, the Ghanaian government has reported a decline in outpatient cases from 6.1 million in 2019 to 5.2 million in 2022.

This is only a brief look into some of the successes of global health. Other successes include water sanitation, tuberculosis control, HIV prevention, tobacco control, and so many more. In addition, none of these problems are fully solved; this article merely shines a light on some of the greatest successes. There is still significant work to be done to improve global health and increase global equity. To learn more about global health, visit the United Nations' Sustainable Development Goals.

Advocating for the Future of Public Health

by Aidan Strealy

The concept of "public health" may sound nebulous and vague, but it plays a critical role in safeguarding and promoting the well-being of communities and populations. Under the purview of public health agencies and professionals, this discipline focuses on disease prevention, health promotion, and the mitigation of health risks. Through comprehensive research, surveillance, and intervention strategies, public health agencies work to identify and address health disparities, emerging threats, and environmental factors that can impact community health. With a collective dedication to the greater good, public health professionals work tirelessly to develop policies, implement preventive measures, and educate the public on health matters. Their efforts range from promoting healthy behaviors and vaccinations to ensuring access to quality healthcare services, making public health an indispensable force in fostering healthier societies, and improving the overall quality of life.

Predictably, addressing a topic with as wide a scope as public health means there are numerous challenges to managing it. For instance, pandemics like COVID-19 pose significant threats to public health infrastructure and response mechanisms. The rapid spread of infectious diseases demands swift and coordinated action to lessen their impact, the failure of which can cause harmful effects on a population.

Additionally, addressing the social determinants of health remains a persistent challenge. Disparities in income, education, access to healthcare, and living conditions significantly influence health outcomes and exacerbate inequalities. Moreover, navigating political differences can hinder the implementation of evidence-based public health policies. Differing ideologies, priorities, and approaches to healthcare can impede the development of unified strategies, hindering the effectiveness of public health initiatives. Despite these challenges, public health professionals continue to work diligently to bridge gaps, advocate for equitable healthcare, and develop strategies to effectively address complex health issues.

Developing a robust system to manage public health yields tremendous benefits for society. While hospitals and healthcare clinics are responsive to existing health problems, the focus of public health is to be preventative of potential health problems. Advocating for proper handwashing is an example, as the National Institutes of Health found that it had strong protective effects of over 95% against influenza infection. By having schools, workplaces, healthcare centers, and government agencies utilize efficient handwashing, influenza's spread is severely limited. And from an economic perspective, Public Health also yields benefits for societies as healthier people are more productive. In fact, Harvard University reports that since healthier people tend to plan for the future, better health results in higher savings rates. A predictive model presented by Walden University estimates that by spending $10 per person on community health programs, the US government could save $16 billion in the long run.

Naturally, these benefits make supporting public health appear logical. However, some believe that taking preventative measures in one area detracts from addressing current issues in another. This, therefore, necessitates the advocacy of public health. One strategy involves engaging policymakers and rallying their support for public health initiatives. By highlighting the benefits and positive impact of these initiatives on communities, public health advocates can influence policymakers to allocate resources, enact legislation, and prioritize public health funding. Another effective approach is forging relationships between public health agencies, healthcare providers, and community organizations. Collaborating and coordinating among these entities can amplify the impact of interventions, ensure efficient resource allocation, and promote community engagement.

The only cost to public health is the effort and funds put forward to continue its development. Aside from the benefits it can bring in the arena of healthcare and preventative measures, the economic impacts of investing in public health would save an enormous amount of money. In the aftermath of the COVID-19 pandemic, the world was forced to learn about the importance of protecting public health. Rather than returning to business as usual in the years following, it makes far more sense to take advantage of this generation's heightened awareness and push for a stronger, more dedicated focus on public health. This way communities will not be caught unaware the next time a health crisis arises and will instead be prepared on both an individual and community level.

What We Need from Our Public Health System

by Bob Kieserman

Throughout the book, we have presented some of the major issues that our public health system is facing right now. As we look to the future, there are many issues that are still not resolved and need more attention.

Women's Health

One of the greatest issues that is facing our country's public health is how to better take care of pregnant women. Initiatives to make pregnancy care and maternal care available to all women, regardless of their race, ethnic group, or financial situation, is imperative. At the same time, all women need to have the opportunity to be screened for gynecological issues and there can be no discrimination of care because of an inability to pay. Mental wellness for all women is also a priority to eliminate unnecessary cases of depression, addiction, and substance abuse. As we have often stated throughout the book, the access to all healthcare services needs to available to all women.

Mental Health

Another major issue that needs to be addressed and proactively implemented is to make sure that all American, regardless of their age, race, gender, sexual orientation, and financial situation have equal access to mental health services.

The government and the nonprofit sector needs to collaborate on creating mental health urgent care centers and outreach facilities where anyone who needs guidance or help in receiving therapy can go and receive it without any stigma attached. Mental healthcare can no longer be a privilege. It must become a right.

Nutrition
Good health begins with healthy eating and wellness. Food deserts need to be eliminated, and all Americans need to have the ability to access healthy food through food banks, neighborhood grocery stores, and food trucks going into neighborhoods with plant-based food, rich in vegetables, healthy protein choices, and fruit. At the same time, the public health system needs to address obesity and provide education and coaching to those who need it, along with organized free exercise programs and recreation opportunities year round. This must become a priority. Hunger and the lack of healthy food choices need to be eliminated.

Aging
As folks live longer, the public health system needs to implement formal programs that offer caregiving to those who cannot afford to pay for it privately. We need programs that offer socialization for the elderly, food for those who cannot afford to buy it, and public housing to provide dignified places to live for those who can no longer afford to maintain a home or apartment. We need to have better regulation of nursing homes and assisted living centers, as well as public adult care centers with qualified caregivers. Our elderly need to become another priority for the public health system guaranteeing that all senior citizens, whether independent or not, can live the best quality of life possible.

Preventive Health

Finally, our public health system needs to continue to be the leading proponent of protecting people from communicable diseases and helping all Americans to stay as healthy as possible. This includes offering free vaccines, extensive patient education, free health screenings, safer neighborhoods, and medical care for those who cannot pay for it privately. While our Medicare and Medicaid systems may need to change as the population changes, the public health system needs to be the country's main source and advocate for better health for all Americans, with no American left behind.

ABOUT THE AUTHORS

Brianna Allison graduated from Duquesne University with a Bachelor's degree in Multiplatform Journalism and one in Public Relations. Brianna has a strong passion for storytelling and loves being a part of a media-enriched environment. She has worked in broadcast journalism, social media, and print journalism in the past. As part of the executive team of The National Library of Patient Rights and Advocacy, Bri served as Managing Editor of *Today's Patient,* she was a Senior Anchor for the broadcast team, and also served as Director of Communications. She is now a digital producer for a television network affiliate.

Hugo Amador is an undergraduate student at Cornell University currently studying cellular & molecular biology, journalism, and Latin American studies. He is the recipient of prestigious and competitive academic fellowships, such as the Cornell Commitment Fellowship, and is the founder of Hugo's Movement, a not-for-profit that advocates for the access to equitable healthcare, education, and liberty of victims of war and gang violence, primarily immigrant children and adolescents.

Olivia Arkell is a recent graduate from Hamline University who studied psychology, philosophy, neuroscience, and political science. She has a strong interest in biomedical ethics and the psychotherapeutic value of psychedelics. Olivia is always looking for ways she can expand her understanding on how we can transform the way we treat mental illness in the clinical setting. She demonstrates this passion through researching and interpreting literature then translating it into a short article/blog form that is easy, reliable, and comprehensible for the general public to read. Olivia joined the editorial team at Today's Patient in spite of initiating important conversations on topics related to wellness, mental health, neuroscience, and psychology and educating people on patient rights and advocacy.

Dima Bischoff-Hashem is an accomplished undergraduate at Rutgers University pursuing a double major in public health and computer science. She interned with The Power of the Patient last summer, and she is particularly interested in healthcare policy and affordability in healthcare. Last semester, She worked in a lab in her school's department of cell biology and neuroscience, researching treatments for traumatic brain injuries. She also interned with three social work professors at Rutgers to contribute research for their publication on environmental justice. Dima hopes to take classes in addiction policy and public health law and aims to affect policy change in her career. Dima was one of the authors of our book, *Reasonable Expectations: The Patient Side of Patient Centered Care.*

Kealan Connors has always wanted to help people in any way, shape, or form. From a young age, he has always been engaged within his community, from building walking/biking trails in his local parks to helping his friends. This desire led him to pursue a degree in communications from Southern Oregon University. He also holds an associate's degree in Arts from Rouge Community College.

Angela DeMondo I completed my undergraduate studies at Arizona State University, earning a Bachelor of Science degree in Health Sciences with honors. Her interest in healthcare and patient advocacy was sparked upon discovering the prevalence of hypertension throughout my familial lineage. Furthermore, as a college student, she initiated the Wasted Wednesday Campaign with the aim of raising awareness about the escalating issue of single-use mask pollution and providing education on the appropriate utilization and disposal of masks amidst the COVID-19 pandemic. In addition, she has authored a policy brief that tackles the spike in the single-use plastic dilemma amidst the Covid-19 outbreak. This paper aims to provide a comprehensive analysis, explanation, and proposed alternatives to address the issue of single-use plastics within the context of the State of Arizona.

Alix Greenblatt has a Bachelor of Arts Degree with a major in International Relations from the State University of New York at New Paltz. She is currently working on completing her MPH program, as well as a certificate in Global Health Studies with the University at Albany. Her goals are to one day work toward improving health rights for women, improve efforts for wildlife/environmental conservation, and to work toward ending the stigma behind mental illness.

Teri Halliwell is a talented writer and broadcaster who earned her undergraduate degree in Journalism from The American College of Greece, and her Masters of Fine Arts in Creative Writing from the University of San Francisco. Teri is an inventive storyteller with a passion for moving audiences to action through her writing. She is a member of the International Association of Professional Writers and Editors, and is a popular host with The Power of the Patient Project. She is also a member of the editorial staff of our online magazine, Today's Patient, where she writes insightful articles on patient-centered health and wellness.

Bob Kieserman is the Executive Director of The Power of the Patient Project: The National Library of Patient Rights and Advocacy, and publisher of *Today's Patient* and this book. Now retired, for over 35 years, he was a professor of healthcare administration and medical ethics and a healthcare consultant. He is the author of over 300 articles and five books on provider/patient relations, managing the private healthcare practice, and patient rights. Bob is both a medical librarian and a medical sociologist and resides near Philadelphia.

Ruby Laine (she/her) is a current undergraduate student at The George Washington University pursuing a Bachelor's of Science in Public Health. She is passionate about improving health outcomes for underserved communities, families, and children. She wishes to assist in expanding access to healthcare and promoting healthy lifestyle behaviors. She has previously worked as an advocate for constituents and the community with the NYC Department of Emergency Management as well as the NYC City Council in District 2. As a Senior Contributor of *Today's Patient*, Ruby focuses on reaching out to wider audiences, to spread awareness of health concerns and improve health literacy.

Caitlin Laska is from Boston and is currently a student at Northeastern University. She is studying public health and international affairs, with a focus on health disparities, education, and global health. She speaks Spanish and Portuguese. She has taught English as a second language to refugees in Jordan, and she has studied abroad in Greece, UAE, Jordan, Egypt, and Ghana during her undergrad years. She currently works as a co-op at Harvard Medical School.

Elizabeth Linden is a retired special education teacher with 25 years of experience. She has a bachelor's degree in Special Education and a master's degree in Health Psychology. Liz has been an advocate for the educational needs of special education students throughout her career as well as an advocate for her own medical needs as a person with a rare headache disorder. Liz is also a Senior Anchor with The Power of the Patient Project, and her interviews are featured throughout our digital library.

Liya Moges is a passionate and dedicated junior studying Biomedical Science, Business, and Law at Georgia State University. She works at Emory University Hospital supporting nurses and physicians on a Complex Medicine floor and uses this opportunity to shadow different physicians in different specialties. In her goal to educate the public about health issues and equal access to care, Liya joined Today's Patient to address topics such as health and wellness, public health, and diversity inclusion in medicine.

Ashley Mui is a junior at UCLA with an interest in medical ethics and healthcare law. She has previously performed research as part of NYU's Emerging Leaders Program. She assessed risk factors for respiratory health in NYC's low-income communities and engineered a particulate matter filtration design for the NYC MTA. She is interested in the sociocultural factors affecting healthcare access, particularly amongst underserved communities.

Emma Nolan is a graduate of Pennsylvania State University with Bachelor's of Science in Biobehavioral Health and minor in Rehabilitation and Human Services. She recently earned a Master's of Public Health with a concentration in Health Systems Organization and Policy from The Penn State College of Medicine. She is currently Manager of Government Relations and Health Initiatives at The Arc of Pennsylvania.

Elika Oakley is a recent graduate from the University of Redlands. She has two Bachelors of Arts in Health, Medicine, and Society & Public Policy. Elika strives to dismantle health disparities and stigmatization by providing information and strategies to address the root cause of health complications. She believes that health is a basic human right and everyone should have equitable access to quality healthcare. Aside from being an advocate for health equity, she is an avid baker, an above average roller skater, and a Bay Area native.

Courtney Pokallus is a graduate of Arcadia University's School of Global Business with a degree in Healthcare Administration and a minor in Global Public Health. At Arcadia, she was a member of the swimming team. She is very interested in healthcare and the healthcare system in the United States. During the summer of 2022, Courtney served as the Associate Director of Provider Outreach and Education at The Power of the Patient Project.

Michelle Powell is an undergraduate student at Michigan State University majoring in Human Biology with plans to become a physician or a physician assistant. She is passionate about writing stories to help people. This led her to join her school's Her Campus chapter. With her passion for journalism, Michelle joined the *Today's Patient* team to focus on medicine and medical issues to help patients better understand how to navigate the healthcare system.

Cori Ritchey is a Washington D.C. native newly transplanted to the Boston area, expected to graduate from Emerson College in 2022 with a Masters in Journalism. She is a graduate of Penn State University with a bachelors of science in Kinesiology. Through her experience working on the frontlines of health care, led by a love for reading, writing, and public speaking, Cori became a health and science reporter to shed light on these issues.

Anooshka Shukla has a Bachelors of Science and with a major in Public Health from Massachusetts College of Pharmacy and Health Sciences (MCPHS) and is currently pursuing Masters of Public Health from the same university, with plans to graduate this summer. She worked as a Teaching Fellow for Citizen School in Boston, MA which works to help inner city students achieve their full potential. She assisted senior citizens in an adult day care center providing health care information. Anooshka also volunteered in a local pharmacy assisting with logistics and customer service. Being passionate about public health, Anooshka is always excited to empower patients, especially in mental health area. Anooshka was one of the authors of our book, *Reasonable Expectations: The Patient Side of Patient Centered Care.*

Maia Signore is a talented writer who attends Arcadia University. Maia has distinguished herself in the sport of competitive swimming, and has devoted much her writing to the current issues in public health.

Emily Sokol, MPH graduated from Brown University with a master's degree in public health and Boston College with a bachelor's degree in English. Emily has worked across the public health field in patient education, journalism and event organizing, government contracting, and care management. Blending her passions for public health and writing, Emily helped The Power of the Patient Project raise awareness of the public health issues that affect us all.

Aidan Strealy is a senior at the University of Redlands in southern California. After completing his studies, he will earn a Biology degree with a minor in English Literature, which he hopes to apply to his career in pursuit of becoming a medical writer. In addition to running for his University's Cross Country and Track and Field teams, Aidan works as a Resident Assistant. The Power of the Patient project drew his attention because while healthcare is an enormous industry in the US, there aren't many opportunities for patients to be educated on how the system works. Aidan is working with us this summer to contribute to the growing body of research and to use his writing background to make medicine and healthcare less daunting for patients.

Kylie Tangonan is a student at Barnard College of Columbia University studying Medical Anthropology. She is passionate about sharing stories and resources that resonate with patients by exploring the ever changing and dynamic fields of medicine, science, public health, and beyond.

Faalik Zahra studies neuroscience and journalism at the University of Cincinnati and plans on becoming a physician. She has always had a strong inclination towards writing and sharing stories which have led her to pursue a journalism degree as well as founding an online media portal, Bearcat Voice. As a Senior Contributor, Faalik combines her passion for writing and her interest in medicine to explain medical issues to patients in a way they can clearly understand.

Index

T

Made in the USA
Middletown, DE
05 October 2023

40326302R00126